CANCER AND COMMON SENSE

COMBINING SCIENCE AND NATURE TO CONTROL CANCER

by

DOUGLAS BRODIE, M.D., with
MICHAEL L. CULBERT DSc

WINNING PUBLICATIONS
2372 Leibel St.
White Bear Lake, MN 55110

Copyright ©1997 by Dr. Douglas Brodie

First Edition: August, 1997

Printed in the United States of America

ISBN: 1-884367-03-8

DEDICATION

This book is dedicated to John A. Richardson, M.D. and Michael L. Culbert, D.Sc., two people who have had major influences on two important aspects of my life and the directions it has taken. These two individuals have also had a major influence in bringing forth innovative methods of treatment in this country and in other parts of the world. Each has contributed hugely toward establishing freedom of choice in medicine, particularly in the treatment of cancer.

Dr. John A. Richardson was a dedicated physician who was a true pioneer and fearless combatant in the continuing war between the proponents of freedom and those who have used oppressive and dictatorial methods to suppress freedom of choice. This courageous man was one of the early casualties in that war, first being subjected to a lengthy, costly and humiliating trial, then losing his medical license in the state of California, and finally making the ultimate sacrifice -- his life. His mistake, from the point of view of the medical establishment, was his choice to be an advocate of the forbidden laetrile, long before most people had even heard of this natural substance and its possible usefulness in the control of cancer. I was privileged to be associated with Dr. Richardson for 8 of the last 10 years of his life, and it was largely due to his influence that I made the decision to pursue the same truthful and humanitarian course as he had, in spite of all odds and all of the hazards that such pursuit would entail.

My co-author, Michael Culbert has been an essential part of this endeavor, as a profound source of knowledge as well as extensive experience in writing about difficult medical subjects with political overtones, especially those involving cancer alternatives. I am indebted to him for the impetus and encouragement to continue when at times my determination would sag and the pressures of my medical practice would take precedence over the book project.

A lifelong journalist, Culbert has been involved for 25 years as an activist in the fight for medical freedom of choice. He has served as chairman of the Committee for Freedom of Choice in Cancer Therapy, Inc., and remains as editor of its publication _The Choice_. He has served as founder and president of the International Council for Health Freedom. Mr. Culbert was instrumental in the formation of the Office of Alternative Medicine (OAM) within the National Institutes of Health. He is the director of information for

American Biologics-Mexico and research writer for the related Bradford Research Institute.

This widely traveled, award winning California journalist was a key figure in helping to secure "decriminalization" of laetrile in over 20 states in the '70's and '80's, and his first book, *Vitamin B17: Forbidden Weapon Against Cancer*, is considered a classic in this area.

Culbert is also the author of the following books:

How You Can Beat the Killer Diseases
What the Medical Establishment Won't Tell You that Could Save Your Life
Freedom from Cancer
Live Cell Therapy
Live Cell Therapy for the 21st Century
AIDS: Hope, Hoax and Hoopla
AIDS: Terror, Truth and Triumph
CFS: Conquering the Crippler
Nutritional and Herbal Factors in the Prevention and Management of Cancer
Medical Armageddon, a 4 volume work, currently being revised to a single volume

Culbert has also authored dozens of articles in magazines, periodicals and newspapers in the field of integrative medicine. His career in journalism has included the editing of newspapers in Berkeley, California, and serving as foreign correspondent for Time/Life and for NBC.

His depth of knowledge and journalistic experience has been indispensable in creating this work.

Douglas Brodie, M.D.

TABLE OF CONTENTS

From the desk of . . .
James W. Forsythe, M.D.

It has been my privilege and honor to know Dr. Douglas Brodie, both professionally and personally for the past fifteen years. As a Board certified internist and medical oncologist with a strong background in Anatomic and Clinical Pathology (Board eligible), and also a current background in Medical Gerontology, I have over my 24 years of practice in Reno, Nevada, been exposed to a large number of patients who were treated by Dr. Brodie and whom I have witnessed firsthand remarkable and astonishing improvements in their course of cancer longevity, both in the area of prolonged remissions and I dare say cures who by conventional standards should have long ago become mortality statistics.

Many of these patients did not have the "benefits" of conventional surgery, radiation therapy, or chemotherapy, but rather on their own volition with freedom of medical choice elected to take alternative medical treatments. Although Dr. Brodie has not had formal training in Medical Oncology, he has a great depth of knowledge in this field having practiced in the area of alternative cancer therapies for the past 25 years.

In addition to being an internist, Dr. Brodie is certified in homeopathy in the State of Nevada and holds a current license to practice both conventional allopathic medicine in this state and homeopathy. Like Dr. Brodie, I attended a Top 10 medical school, the University of California in San Francisco, and I graduated in the top 20% of my class. During the four years that I attended the University of California in San Francisco Medical Center, I did not hear the word homeopathy mentioned once. Formal teaching in nutrition, vitamin and mineral therapy, immune dysfunction, chronic viral illnesses, environmental toxins, and preventative medicine occupied a very small portion of the four year curriculum, and I dare say less than two hours of formal teaching in these areas was given. Most of my education in these extremely important areas of modern medicine came through my interest in preventative and holistic medicine which I acquired after my internship, and my experience while serving with the U.S. Army in the Republic of South Vietnam as a major in the U.S. Army Medical Core.

During my residency and fellowship years in San Francisco, I became further interested in looking at alternatives to toxic *chemotherapy and radiation therapy. I witnessed innumerable incidences of patients being put through exhaustive, toxic, disabling, chemotherapy when there was no hope in sight, and when the disease process (namely their terminal cancer) was already an established fact. When I began practicing in the State of Nevada in 1974, I was fortunate to have picked a state which was tolerant of alternative medical practices, namely homeopathy and naturopathy.*

Over the past score of years, I have personally witnessed innumerable successes with alternative therapies and have become singularly impressed of the body's self-healing ability and the many unknown factors which go into the healing process of which conventional medicine has little or no knowledge. These include mind/body interactions, effective positive thinking, denial, prayer, hope, and an intense drive on the part of individual patients to seek out and educate themselves on natural healing methods. To seek out and earnestly form a partnership with physicians who are willing to give them the time they need to develop a personal strategy against their disease using all forms of natural therapy, either with or without the addition of conventional therapies.

Dr. Brodie's book <u>Cancer and Common Sense</u> is extremely educating and will make an excellent reference for any physician or patient interested in these areas. He covers not only the field of conventional cancer therapy and its problems, but also the integrated therapies sighting specific case examples. He talks about his experience with alternative therapies and patient successes. He goes into great detail on the politics of medicine and the political, medical, pharmaceutical cancer treatment complex which dominates conventional medicine, and even covers in an extremely informative way the immune system and immune modulation, a chapter I found extremely interesting. He talks about the theories behind anti-oxidants, vitamin, herbal, and mineral therapies as well as newer therapies on the cutting edge of cancer treatment. Treatment modalities which are virtually unknown and unexplored by conventional medical oncologists. He also talks about mind/body interaction and the concept of wellness.

Dr. Brodie's work and dedication to his art and science has not come without personal sacrifice. He has been attacked relentlessly by State Board of Medical Examiners, especially in the State of California and literally has had to face numerous trials and threat of license forfeiture because of his activities. Over the years, personally knowing Dr. Brodie and seeing his patients, I have not seen a single case of adverse treatment outcome in terms of toxicity, severe morbidity, or death from any of his natural treatments. Dr. Andrew Wiel, a highly respected conventional and alternative medicine physician, who is Harvard trained and heads the Department of Integrative Medicine at the University of Arizona, would undoubtedly feel as I do that Dr. Brodie is the model of the physician of the new millennium. This model portrays a physician who is not only well learned in conventional medicine, but also has a grasp of natural healing of nutrition, vitamin, mineral, and herbal remedies, folk remedies, naturopathy, homeopathy, acupuncture, and all the other modalities of holistic medicine.

The type of medicine that Dr. Brodie practices is the antithesis of the New Age managed care medicine which simply stated is high volume, low quality medicine where quantity is what counts. Physicians are rewarded both monetarily and through ranking if they see patients rapidly in high volume, order less tests, prescribe fewer medicines, and request less consultations. In other words, they never really address the patients' true problems. And God forbid they ever try to treat something in the gray area of medicine such as immune dysfunction diseases, chronic viral illnesses, incurable neurologic or arthritic conditions, or advanced neoplastic diseases.

After all, homeopathy is over 200 years old where as American medicine as we know it today is only 150 years old. Homeopathy is used by over 500 million people throughout the world and in reality is the predominant form of medical care. Therefore, it should not be labeled alternative, but on a world scale is the conventional form of medicine. It is practiced on all continents and is especially popular in England, the Orient, and India. In England, it receives royal patronage.

It is unfortunate to state, however, that we have not come that far in our tolerance of alternative medical practices. For instance, in the 19th Century, an allopathic or conventional physician could have his license revoked or be totally ostracized by his profession just by consulting with a homeopathic physician. In the early 20th Century, the State Board of Medical Examiners who saw their role as protectors of the public "medical standard" were highly prejudiced against any form of alternative medical care. Alternative medicine as Dr. Brodie clearly states in his book, and as reported by the New England Journal of Medicine, is used in some degree by at least one third of our population. In other countries such as Europe and

Australia, as much as 50% of the population routinely uses alternative care. Despite its widespread use, I continually see patients who tell me that their own doctors will not discuss alternative medicine and berate them for even bringing the subject up. In some cases, I have been told that patients have been dismissed from practices by telling their doctors they use alternative medical treatment.

I feel that Dr. Brodie's book will go a long way to help shed the old prejudices and stereotypes. It will give notice that our nation's health is not just in the hands or jurisdiction of conventional medicine, and that alternative medical practitioners including health food distributors, educators, nutritionists, dieticians, naturopaths, acupuncturists, and oriental medicine practitioners should be valued for their expertise and input. And that conventional medicine will only gain and prosper by the richness and depth of the knowledge gained from the understanding of alternative therapies.

I heartily recommend this book for any physician or alternative medicine practitioner, and to the lay public or anyone interested in taking hold of their own health and realizing that we have only one body. We must treat it wisely and that if illness does strike, it is best to use the best of both sides of medicine, namely conventional and alternative treatments.

James W. Forsythe, M.D.

From the desk of . . .
Timothy W. Fraser, D.D.S.

In the early 1980's I saw Dr. Brodie for symptoms of heavy metal toxicity, which he diagnosed through a simple urine test. Actually, it was not really that simple because three previous physicians had missed the correct diagnosis before Dr. Brodie, realizing that I worked with mercury, looked in my mouth to see the color of my gums. True mercury toxicity gives the gum tissue a distinct color.

During the next few months, I had two chelating sessions each week with Dr. Brodie as he followed my mercury levels into a safe zone. During these three hour sessions I had opportunity to speak with many of Dr. Brodie's patients. They all loved Dr. Brodie, and for good reason. Many of these individuals had become healthy, well-functioning people who had been previously condemned to death as "terminal patients" by conventional oncologists. Others had been condemned to the mutilation of conventional surgery, radiation and chemotherapy,. These patients sought Dr. Brodie's care, either initially as an alternative to conventional therapy, or, more often, secondarily after orthodox methods had failed.

In 1992, at age 80, my mother was diagnosed with breast cancer. Her long-time physician warned her that if she did not submit herself to surgery, radiation and chemotherapy, it would mean certain death. Wisely and courageously, she refused these therapies and was treated by Dr. Brodie. Today she is very much alive, healthy and vital.

My experience with Dr. Brodie is one that I have long wished the entire world could share. In his book, <u>Cancer and Common Sense,</u> Dr. Brodie shows that it is possible to erase the terror associated with cancer. Dr. Brodie is a humble, wise man, with a special gift for humanity, if only fear can be given up long enough to allow receptivity of his ideas for positive change.

Timothy W. Fraser, B.S., M.A., D.D.S.

From the desk of . . .
Frank Shallenberger, M.D.

<u>Cancer and Common Sense</u> is an important book. Important because unlike so many other physicians, who are strictly vested in either an alternative or a conventional approach to cancer treatment, Dr. Brodie has found a common sense, common ground perspective that gives his patients the best of both worlds. His heroic battles with the California Medical Board serve to underscore the sad fact that when it comes to medicine, America is clearly <u>**not**</u> the land of the free.

Frank Shallenberger, M.D.

INTRODUCTION

At the beginning of this century, only one American in 30 was afflicted with cancer. Today more than one out of three Americans have or will have cancer at some time in his or her life lifetime.

By the end of this century, at the present rate of increase, it will be closer to one out of two — *half* the population of this country. The old excuse that we are living longer — long enough to develop cancer — is no longer valid, because the disease is being diagnosed at younger and younger ages.

The onset of most cancers occurs between the ages of 40 and 60 years and it has been my observation that with some of the major cancers, such as those involving breast, pancreas, and colon, I am now seeing more and more younger victims of this disease than I did years ago.

While the *rate* of cancer occurrence has increased dramatically over the past century, the *length of survival* has declined drastically — this, despite our vaunted technology and buckets of money thrown at the problem. Some honest physicians and researchers now acknowledge that we are indeed losing the battle. Even as new anti-cancer drugs and new techniques are developed, survival rates for the major cancers continue to decline at an increasing rate.

This reality was only partly mitigated by the National Cancer Institute's announcement in late 1996 that for the first time actual cancer fatality rates were beginning to turn down (a drop of 2.6% between 1991 and 1995) even while rates of incidence kept spiralling upward.

Despite many years of intensive research, intensified since the "War on Cancer" was declared 26 years ago, establishment medicine has not come much closer to understanding the basic underlying cause or causes of cancer. More importantly, neither has it come much closer to finding safe and effective treatments.

The longer-term results of conventional treatment of cancer remain disheartening to patients and physicians alike.

While most oncologists are sincere in their desire to do the best for their patients, they are confined to "approved" drugs, procedures and protocols, and dare not venture beyond these narrow limitations for fear of enormous pressure from their peers, as well as government sanctions and penalties which are designed to enforce conformity and which could result in loss of their medical licenses. Physicians are perhaps more sensitive to such pressure and sanction than members of any other profession, since their very professional survival depends upon acceptance by the medical community and, worse still, upon compliance with one overbearing government agency or another.

As discussed in this book, it has been the pharmaceutical industry which has been the primary force in maintaining the status quo of American medicine. By providing huge grants to most of the major research institutions, the pharmaceutical complex exerts enormous influence on the direction of research in this country. *All* advertising in all of the hundreds of our medical journals comes from the giants of the pharmaceutical industry, thus imposing upon the medical profession the rigid and unchallengeable school of thought sometimes referred to as allopathy.

Add to this monopoly of thought the power of the federal government and you have a nearly impenetrable barrier to new ideas in medicine. This unfortunate barrier seems to be more unyielding and more stifling to innovation in the field of cancer than in any other branch of medicine.

This static condition of cancer therapy has not gone unnoticed by the many victims of cancer, who are seeking alternative solutions in ever greater numbers. Some estimates suggest that the seekers of alternative care (not just for cancer) may run as high as 40% to 50% of the total patient population. Of course, most of these patients continue to have conventional care, but often in conjunction with some degree of complementary, alternative or integrative medical care.

This book will explore many of the reasons, political, economic and otherwise, which have led to this impasse, and will discuss many of the alternatives available, either as enhancers of traditional methods, or even, in some cases, as viable methodologies by themselves.

My co-author and I expose new ideas and proposals — not just our own — regarding the basic nature and causation of cancer. We do not claim to have all of the answers to this problem, of course, and assuredly make no claims to having a cure of cancer. But certainly the application of some common sense and honest observation can do no harm and will hopefully help to make some progress in changing the direction of research, prevention and treatment of a disease which has become an American nightmare.

This book is a review of my clinical experience in the management of many cancer patients for over 20 years, applying knowledge gleaned from many sources, many ages and many countries, along with the knowledge acquired from direct observation in caring for these patients. Included are a few case histories which demonstrate not only the potential for long-term survival with alternative methods, but also the possibilities for enhancement of conventional methods with the addition of proper diet, specific nutritional supplementation, and certain non-toxic substances, together with appropriate psychological support.

Even the acknowledgment by conventional oncologists and radiation therapists that such supplementation can increase the effectiveness of their methods of treatment would be, in our opinion, a boon to their practices, and most certainly a welcome benefit to their patients. Besides boosting the effectiveness of orthodox treatment, proper supplementation and non-toxic methods or modalities have another important influence on the patient's well-being: they protect against the adverse side effects of conventional chemotherapy and radiation, often eliminating them altogether.

One would think that mainstream physicians would be interested in securing these benefits for their patients, but the suggestion of such has often been met with rejection and even hostility.

One of the criticisms we in alternative medicine frequently hear from our conventional colleagues is that "there is no documentation" that any of the unconventional methods have any proven effectiveness. In this book are some 180 references, many in "peer-reviewed" journals read by or available to traditional practitioners. For more documentation, the reader is referred to other books, such as *Cancer Therapy* by Ralph W. Moss Ph.D, which contains over 1000 such references.

In this book, we explore a wide variety of substances, mostly natural, which have the capacity to modify or inhibit the progression of cancer, as well as substances which appear to be able to prevent its development. The importance of a healthy immune system is stressed, along with suggestions as to how this can be maintained, usually with some fairly simple changes in one's lifestyle.

While this is not a "do-it-yourself" handbook for treating cancer, one of the important messages we wish to convey is that the cancer patient must be an active participant in his or her own health care. We all still need doctors, of course, but the cancer victim is encouraged to explore all avenues, rather than to be confined to conventional methods alone. Much can be done to improve the odds against developing cancer and the chances of surviving it once it has developed.

This is our message of hope.

Douglas Brodie, M.D.
Winter 1996/1997

Chapter I
'INTEGRATIVE' THERAPY
Turning Cancer Around

TWENTY YEARS CONTROLLING MULTIPLE CANCERS

It was on May 5, 1977, that a 49-year-old male physicist, Robert Fowler, who was working at a high-stress US Navy weapons facility, came to my office in Tahoe City CA with the following history:

The prior August (1976) he had developed what seemed to a boil on the back of his lower neck. Since it didn't just "go away," he decided to visit a local physician who allegedly "popped" the boil. It drained pus for three months thereafter.

In mid-January 1977, and now suspecting something a little more threatening might be involved, he had been seen at a tumor clinic in Pasadena, California.

Experts there noted that there was a persistent draining abscess at the rear base of the neck — and that Mr. Fowler had developed an enlarged lymph node above the right collar bone, or at the forward base of the neck, which had been enlarging since September. The mass by this time measured 6 cm. wide.

Doctors there took cultures of the draining lesion and, detecting two bacteria, *Aerobacter aerogenes* and *Enterococcus*, started him on a course of antibiotics. These seemed to help some, but the infection persisted.

On January 28, a needle biopsy — removing a small sliver of tissue through a needle for the purpose of establishing a diagnosis — was carried out at the Pasadena clinic on the mass in front of the neck. This proved to be cancerous — specifically "squamous cell carcinoma." At the same time, a biopsy was taken from the chronically draining lesion in the lower back of the neck.

This was negative for malignancy at first, but subsequent biopsies finally revealed that it contained the same type of cancer as the tissue that had been taken from the node in the right frontal neck area. The latter was considered to be *metastatic* cancer (that which has spread to a distant area from the original or "primary" site), and the open lesion in the back of the neck was considered to be the "primary." This diagnosis was confirmed by several qualified pathologists.

Following standard procedures, X-rays of the chest and sinus cavities plus tomograms and esophagrams were carried out to see if there was cancer in these areas. They were accompanied by biopsies of the bronchial tubes, larynx and base of the tongue. All were negative.

The first "orthodox" procedure Robert underwent was then carried out — surgery (called a "wide excision") of the persistently non-healing lesion on the back of the neck.

Unlike many instances, in which oncological surgeons may triumphantly announce that they "got it all" and that removal of the primary tumor somehow can then be equated with the "curing" of cancer, his doctors realized that there already was "metastatic disease" (the cancer had spread) and they thought that the lower margin of the surgical wound might also contain cancer cells.

The cancer experts then went to the next level in orthodox thinking — they suggested localized radiation to be followed by the surgical removal of all lymph nodes on the right side of the neck, a procedure called "radical neck dissection."

On Feb. 18 "deep radiation" of the neck and mediastinum with Cobalt-60 was begun, with 23 treatments taking place over 31 days paralleled by five localized treatments of the original lesion.

During this month or so of therapy the rear lesion gradually healed but had some residual burning from the radiation and there was also some reduction in the frontal mass.

All this was done preliminary to the "radical neck dissection," and during which time Mr. Fowler had plenty of time to think — and learn — about cancer and the essential failure of modern "orthodox" medicine, particularly in spread or metastatic stages of the disease.

Just a few days before the operation was scheduled, Robert called his surgeon and canceled the surgery. The surgeon stated in a letter that he was "terribly distressed" over the patient's decision and that without surgery he had only six months to live or at most a year. Remember that this was in 1977.

Since this patient had learned, perhaps in the nick of time, that there are "alternative" methods available for cancer treatment, if not well known about or recommended by medical orthodoxy, he found out about my practice at Lake Tahoe and arrived on May 5 seeking help.

This was fairly early in my career as a preventive-medicine, holistic and alternative therapy-oriented physician, one of many who over time had turned from standard or "allopathic" practice to these newer and, in our mind, more benign and effective therapies.

I immediately placed him on an immune system-supportive program including intravenous vitamins, minerals, special immune-enhancing substances including thymus gland peptides, and the highly controversial unorthodox anti-cancer drug laetrile, a preparation extracted from apricot seeds and essentially consisting of the chemical amygdalin, which some were calling "Vitamin B17." At the time, laetrile was the center of a white-hot medical controversy in the USA (*see Chapter IX*).

During the course of his three-week stay as an outpatient at my clinic, I referred him to a Reno surgeon and requested a simple surgical removal of the still-present frontal neck node. I had selected this particular surgeon because, unlike so many others, he was more tolerant of "alternative" therapies. But even he would not consider anything less than the radical neck dissection, the very procedure our patient had firmly rejected.

I then discussed with Robert all the "alternative" approaches to this particular problem that I knew about and information on which was available from worldwide research.

We decided to proceed with local injection into the node of a German preparation of proteolytic (protein-digesting) enzymes called Wobe-Mugos. The idea here, advanced decades before, was that proteolytic enzymes are a primary first line of defense against the malignant or cancer process and that such enzymes may help "digest" the protein coating of the cancer cells and expose them to immune system attack as well as engage in some of the attack themselves. This line of research had never been followed up on very seriously in the USA.

Node injections of this preparation were carried out with the accompanying immune-support program of laetrile, oral enzymes, peptides, various nutritional antioxidants and vitamins A, C, E and certain minerals, which themselves often function as antioxidants (*see Chapter VII*).

The first intratumoral Wobe-Mugos injection was on May 22 with 100 mg of the enzyme solution mixed with 2 cc of lidocaine.

Initial measurement of the node before the first injection was 3.8 cm X 3.3 cm. A week later, as anticipated, the node had *increased* to 4.5 cm X 4.0 cm. It was larger because of fluid buildup which, to metabolic therapists, usually means the tumor mass is actually beginning to respond to therapy by way of liquefaction or becoming liquefied.

After another week, "aspiration," or needle puncture and withdrawal under local anesthesia, yielded 3.5 cc. of amber-colored fluid containing white particulate matter. Removal of the fluid reduced the mass to 3.5 X 3.0 cm. We then administered another 100 mg of the enzyme preparation.

Between June 8, 1977, and Jan, 1, 1978, I did weekly injections of the node, each time aspirating fluid before introducing the enzymes, and each time being careful to inject only into the fluid-containing cavity created by the enzymes.

While the size of the node fluctuated during this time, the general direction was a *decrease* in size of the mass.

Over a six-month period I sent samples of aspirated fluid, drained from the mass, to a pathologist. The pathological examination of this liquid showed dramatic changes from many malignant cells at first to fewer and fewer cells until, on Jan. 3, 1978, no such cells were observable at all. And the size of the mass had reduced to 1.5 cm X 1.5 cm.

Copies of the pathologist's report and letter are shown in Figs. 1 through 4 primarily to illustrate not only that cancer cells were indeed not present in the last specimen, but also to show the hostile attitude of the pathologist over the fact that this aspirated material had changed from highly malignant to non-malignant, from containing many cancer cells to containing none. The pathologist was obviously unhappy about this. Why?

Over the years I have observed this attitude rather frequently on the part of physicians wedded to mainstream thought — namely, anger and hostility toward those of us who have applied unconventional treatment modalities, even when — sometimes *especially* when — those modalities are successful. This seems incredible to most of my patients and others who have observed this phenomenon, since the

MML/Solano Laboratories

2920 TELEGRAPH AVENUE
BERKELEY, CALIFORNIA 94705
(415) 549-1823

Fowler, Robert

Date sampled down | Age

5/31/77

Date Recd | Lab #

6/2/77 | 77-S-429

Referred by

W. Douglas Brodie, M.D.
P.O. Box 12
Tahoe City, CA. 95730

ATTENTION

Clinical Data:

Source of specimen: From lymph node.

Gross Description: The specimen consists of fragments of tissue too small to pick up with forceps. Specimen centrifuged and cell block made.

Microscopic Examination: The cell block consists of fragments of tissue that are completely squamous cell carcinoma. Most of the cells are keratinizing.

MICROSCOPIC DIAGNOSIS: Keratinizing squamous cell carcinoma.

Grace M. Hyde, M.D.

DATE REPORTED 6/6/77

HAROLD M. MALKIN, M.D., Director

Figure 1: Material aspirated from lymph node on May 31, 1977

W. Douglas Brodie, M.D.
P.O. Box 12
Tahoe City, CA. 95730

ATTENTION:

MML/Solano Laboratories

2820 TELEGRAPH AVENUE
BERKELEY, CALIFORNIA 94705
(415) 549-1823

Source of specimen: Supraclavicular.

Clinical Data:
—

Gross Description:

Microscopic Examination:

Both a nucleopore and cell block of the fluid received have been made. The nucleopore preparation shows many cells, but primarily multinucleated foreign body type giant cells, foamy histiocytic cells, crystalline debris and chronic inflammatory cells. The cell block sections show primarily similar cells but in addition a few neoplastic squamous cells. The giant cells and foamy histiocytes are seen quite commonly as a reaction to spilled keratinous debris in ruptured sebaceous cysts. In fact so much of the cellular material is of this type that a review of the original material was made to be certain the original material had not been over diagnosed. Following this, a renewed search was made of the present material and this disclosed a few isolated neoplastic squamous cells.

MICROSCOPIC DIAGNOSIS:

Squamous carcinoma cells.

Grace M. Hyde, M.D.

DATE REPORTED 9/15/77

HAROLD M. MALKIN, M.D. Director

Figure 2: Material aspirated from lymph node September 6, 1977

No. _____ Given / Robert _____

MML Solano Laboratories

2800 TELEGRAPH AVENUE
BERKELEY, CALIFORNIA 94705
415-549-1623

W. Douglas Brodie, M.D.
P.O. Box 12
Tahoe City, CA. 95730

12/5/77

12/7/77   77-S-946

Clinical Data:

Gross Description:

Source of specimen: Right supraclavicular node.

Microscopic Examination:

Multiple sections of the cell block of aspirated material
show a pink staining background of protein aceous material
containing entrapped white blood cells. A nucleopore
preparation was attempted but it rapidly became clogged.
There are red and white blood cells and a few histiocytes.
No neoplastic cells are seen.

Grace M. Hyde, M.D—

DATE REPORTED 12/13/77

Figure 3: Material aspirated from lymph node on December 7, 1977, showing no
neoplastic (cancer) cells.

MML/Solano Laboratories

2920 Telegraph Avenue/Berkeley, CA 94705/(415) 549-1623

December 28, 1977

W. Douglas Brodie, M.D.
P.O. Box 12
Tahoe City, California 95730

Dear Doctor Brodie:

In response to your request to compare the previous specimens on Robert Fowler, I'd be happy to oblige but it is not possible to compare nothing with something. Incidently it would be helpful if you would supply some clinical information on this patient. To this day, we still have no age. What kind of a mass does he have, how long has he had it and what has happened in the past six months since you stuck a needle in it? Is there some reason it cannot be excised? It is difficult to give a consultation (which is what a pathology request means) without any clinical information.

Grace M. Hyde, M.D.

Figure 4: Letter from pathologist responding to my request to compare the last specimen with previous specimens.

physician's goal is supposed to be to heal the sick and relieve suffering. It appears to me that many conventional physicians — because of their training, their confinement to drug-oriented literature, and heavy peer pressure to conform — feel that any information outside their usual sphere must be highly suspect, and even intimidating, because it is a field completely foreign to them.

I also placed Bob Fowler on what I often think of as the main support for the whole program: attention to an anti-cancer diet (emphasizing less animal fat and protein, few or no refined carbohydrates, few or no stimulants, and more natural fruits and vegetables in as nearly a raw or natural a state as possible, and unrefined grains.) This was of course accompanied by numerous nutritional supplements (vitamins, minerals, enzymes, amino acids) and oral laetrile.

I saw him monthly for the next four months, during which he had no injections. Each time the mass was found to be smaller until May 5, 1978, when it could no longer be felt. At the time of each consultation I examined the patient carefully and evaluated his immune system, finding on each occasion both the patient and his immune system to be vigorous and healthy.

I monitored him closely over the next few years as he continued to put ever-greater distance beyond the prediction of certain death between six months and a year by refusing to undergo the radical neck dissection, and never found any recurrence of the lesion in the lower neck. According to "orthodox" thinking, patient Fowler made it through five years virtually symptom-free, which normally means a "cure" in the strange parlance of conventional oncology. Yet he was not "cured" in the full meaning of that very controversial word.

Throughout most of the year 1982, Bob had noted the development of another suspicious sore — this time toward the side of the right eyebrow. Consequently, on Nov. 3, 1982, he came to my office in Incline Village, Nevada, where the lesion was removed under local anesthesia. A pathology report showed it to be "basal cell carcinoma," in standard oncological thought by no means related to the earlier "squamous cell carcinoma," which was no longer present.

Basal cell carcinomas are the common "skin cancers" that many people have and which have been "curable" by simple removal since the days of Hippocrates — if by "curable" one means five years without symptoms and no evidence of metastasis, or spread. Far more lethal is the form of skin-originating cancer called "melanoma."

And, as fate would have it, melanoma turned out to be the very next diagnosis for Bob Fowler — that is, four years later, or on Nov. 26, 1986, when we found a pigmented mole behind the right knee which appeared suspiciously dark and had a small area of spread at its margins.

Following removal under local anesthesia in my office, the lesion turned out, on pathological examination, to be malignant melanoma.

I add here that over the years — and it had now been nine years since Bob Fowler had been diagnosed with metastatic cancer and told of the certainty of death within a year — he had become less strict about following the prescribed immune-supporting diet with supplements which I place patients on. This is a frequent problem in the natural or metabolic management of cancer patients: getting them to stay on a rational eating and supplementary program, especially when all signs and symptoms of cancer seem to have vanished.

I urged him to be more disciplined in both diet and supplements, particularly with vitamin A, which many of us consider to be of utmost importance in the prevention and care of skin cancer.

More than four years passed. At each checkup Bob seemed to be free of the signs and symptoms of melanoma and in ordinarily good health. But was he "cured" of the *malignant process?* Not cured — but certainly "controlled."

At least until Feb. 27, 1990, when during his visit to my office he complained of a crusted lesion or sore on the right side of the upper neck, well above the site of the original lesion we had successfully treated years before. Excision, or surgical removal, of the lesion was then performed. The pathology report this time came back "basal cell carcinoma" — that is, the same "tumor type" as his second diagnosis in 1982. Fortunately, the margins of the new lesions were found to be free of cancer cells. I then issued new orders about strictness of diet and staying on supplements.

I saw Bob briefly during a convention in Pasadena in 1991 and he told me he had been in good health and had no symptoms.

I then lost track of him for five years until, in March 1996, he was finally located by the Cancer Control Society of Los Angeles, an organization which supports alternative cancer therapies and helps cancer patients find appropriate treatment modalities as well as to find other patients who have had success with those modalities.

After this five-year hiatus, Bob came to my office in Reno on June 25, 1996, for a checkup. Other than a whiplash injury of the neck suffered in an auto-bus accident in 1993, his health had been excellent overall for the intervening years. Regular checkups by his local physicians, including blood chemistries, blood counts, chest X-rays, etc. had revealed no abnormalities. Several suspicious skin lesions had appeared between 1993 and 1996 on his chest, arms, and thighs, all successfully removed by the patient, acting on his own, some with a topical herbal preparation — preparation and some with "Efudex" ointment containing 5FU, a common chemotherapy agent.

My examination revealed no evidence of skin lesions or any other abnormalities, other than some limitation of neck movement. An AMAS test (Anti-Malignin Antibody in Serum — *see Appendix*) was carried out and was found to be normal. At the time of this visit, he was 68 years old, retired, living with his wife in Arizona, active, and busy building a barn on his property.

On October 9, 1996, Bob returned to my office for a checkup. All of the treated skin lesions appeared to be well-healed and benign, except for a small suspicious spreading lesion behind the right knee, in the same area as the previously removed melanoma. Because of its location, its spreading nature and because it contained some dark pigment, this lesion was surgically removed in the office under local anesthesia.

Pathology showed this to be a non-malignant or benign fibrohistiocytoma, still another type of skin pathology. This was a pleasant surprise to all concerned because the appearance of the lesion had suggested melanoma.

The case of Bob Fowler is remarkable on a number of fronts:

First, it is of course most notable that as of this writing (fall 1996) we were looking at a well-documented case of a nearly 20-year survival in ordinarily good health in the person of an individual who was told by the "soundest" medical advice at the time (1977) that without radical neck surgery he would be dead in six months to a year.

It is also a statement that "complementary" or "integrative" therapy — which really means any combination that works — needs to be strongly considered as a viable option even by the most recalcitrant orthodox physician. Because, as in this case, localized radiation and surgery were probably appropriate at the time and served a useful purpose, as did the administration of some antibiotics.

What many of us call "metabolic" or "nutritional" therapy, though, probably had the greatest effect: seen in "unorthodox" eyes, it helped protect his immune system against the negative effects of radiation while also building his immune response against the cancer process.

We can also state that the various confirmed diagnoses of this patient over two decades — squamous cell carcinoma followed by basal cell carcinoma followed by melanoma followed by basal cell carcinoma — speak reams about the "unitarian" concept of cancer (*see Chapter IV*) and the notion that, at root, there is an underlying, subclinical malignant process, whatever "tumor types" or "cell lines" may later be diagnosed to fit the standard oncological notion of "hundreds of types of cancer."

The various diagnoses over the years also tend to confirm the concept that cancer, a malignant process of many parts, is never truly "cured" but may undergo long periods of "control." Were I a standard oncologist using the orthodox "gold standard" of five years, I would have to say in his case "cured" basal cell carcinoma twice, squamous cell carcinoma once and melanoma, the deadliest of all, once. Such a statement looks and sounds incredible — because it is.

Perhaps the most remarkable aspect of this remarkable case is the long survival following the proven diagnosis of *metastatic* (spread) cancer without the usual conventional treatment.

Thanks both to the treatment and his own attention to diet and supplements, Robert Fowler has helped keep a malignant process in check — that is, "under control."

And perhaps equal to if not more important than all these factors, in the Fowler case we are presented with the reality of a man who attitudinally got it all together: he gathered the extreme courage and gumption to reject supposedly life-saving radical surgery, studied all he could on his own, adapted to the discipline of diet and supplements and even made a major career leap — he abandoned a well-paying but highly stressful job with a US Navy weapons center and settled for the less-demanding routine of a bus driver.

He became a participant in his own healing process, not a passive recipient of just doing what the doctor said to do. We inculcate this philosophy as an absolute necessity in every case.

He also was happily wedded to a highly supportive wife whom he married shortly after the beginning of his treatment program. To have a loving support mechanism, be it spouse, relative, friend or group, is of enormous importance in healing.

And aspects of the therapy of course vindicate laetrile, enzymes, nutrients, antioxidants, the theory of detoxification and other natural approaches to a disease process against which, as we shall see, US medical orthodoxy has made woefully little progress.

Lastly, in the face of confusion, negative commentary, intimidation and grave predictions, this man was able to make a free choice, at first, even in California — with its harsh restrictions — then in Nevada. And, after carefully and studiously choosing the combinations of modalities he was most comfortable with, he was then able to implement those choices and to freely talk about alternative therapies, not only with me but with a number of other practitioners of similar persuasion. He is happy he made those choices. I am too.

'CURE' ? — A CASE OF TWENTY-YEAR REMISSION OF PANCREATIC CANCER

Mrs. Maria Basic 65, was first seen at the Richardson Clinic in Albany, California, in 1976, following surgery for cancer of the pancreas.

She had developed upper abdominal pain followed by jaundice and had been operated on at a hospital in San Francisco, during which it was found that there was a large malignant tumor involving the head of the pancreas which was considered to be inoperable. Since it was obstructing the common bile duct, jaundice had resulted.

A bypass procedure was carried out which allowed the bile to flow once again through the bile duct into the small intestine, but the tumor itself could not be removed. The jaundice and pain subsided almost immediately after surgery.

Following the operation the patient was started on an intensive intravenous program, consisting of high doses of vitamin C, minerals, B vitamins, potassium, and other non-toxic substances including laetrile, along with immune enhancing polypeptides and oral supplements. She was also started on the low-animal protein, mostly vegetarian Richardson diet, which she followed religiously. Her jaundice cleared promptly following the surgery, and her abdominal pain gradually subsided over a month on this program. Her feeling of well-being also gradually returned.

Some of the original records of this patient are no longer available, but the basic facts remain recorded. The patient was told by the oncologists and surgeons in San Francisco to go home and "get your affairs in order," and that she might have six months to live.

This lady happened to be a very positive individual who was able to view her situation with a hopeful and optimistic attitude. She was also able and willing to make major changes in her lifestyle and eliminate the negative influences in her life situation.

About eight months after the diagnosis of cancer of the pancreas had been made, a repeat CT scan of the abdomen was carried out at the San Francisco hospital. Much to the surprise of all concerned, the tumor had dramatically reduced in size. Of course, during all this time the patient had been dutifully following her immune enhancement program with all of the special supplements, diet, oral laetrile, and peptide injections which were administered in the clinic several times per week.

She remained completely without symptoms over the ensuing months, with a high level of energy and productivity. Approximately 17 months after the initial treatment a CT scan revealed no evidence of tumor!

Maria has been seen infrequently in my office over the years, but phone contact has been maintained at least annually. She continues to obtain some of her supplements from my office in Reno and continues to follow her program.

The last contact was made in September 1996, at which time she was very much alive and well, now age 85 and working as a volunteer in a San Francisco hospital.

DISCUSSION: The remarkable aspect of this case, I believe, is that this lady received no conventional treatment for what is ordinarily considered a particularly difficult and resistant type of cancer. The surgery that was carried out had served to relieve the jaundice only and did not specifically address the cancer. Consequently, much as it may pain the conventional doctors to acknowledge this, the favorable result can be attributed only to natural and non-toxic modalities, including, of course, lifestyle and attitudinal changes.

Though we in the alternative field are always reluctant to use the word "cure," I feel that a 20-year remission comes pretty close. The cancer establishment has arbitrarily set five years as the criterion for its "cures," which many of us in the field of alternative methods feel is far from adequate, though it may be realistic for conventional treatment.

Chapter II
BEST EVIDENCE —
THE PATIENTS THEMSELVES:
'Integrative' Therapies Work

TEN YEARS CONTROLLING LYMPHOMA

I first saw Julian Kosinsky, a then 67-year-old retired fireman, at our facility on June 20, 1986. He had traveled 200 miles to try a new approach to malignant lymphoma, a major killer cancer.

In October the year before he had noticed a lump on the right side of his neck, just beneath the mandible, or jaw bone.

His local physician thought this was probably a salivary gland cyst, so it was simply kept under observation for a month with no change in size or color detected.

In order to be sure, however, an excisional biopsy was ordered. The lump was removed Nov. 12, 1985. Diagnosis: malignant lymphoma.

On about June 5, 1986, he found a second enlarged lymph node or lump below the mandible and just behind the site where the original one had been. "CT" scans of his abdomen and pelvis were negative as were chest X-rays. His local doctors recommended radiation but Mr. Kosinsky decided to try an "alternative" approach, and sought me out that same month.

Other than a 2 cm. by 2 cm. mass beneath the jaw bone on the right side of his neck, his examination was completely normal. Routine laboratory blood work was normal, but his immune function, as determined by the more-or-less controversial darkfield microscopy system, showed a severe lack of activity. (See *appendix*.) This quickly changed with the single injection of a thymus peptide which was followed by a profound increase in white blood cell activity.

I started him out on the basic anti-cancer program and appropriate supplements. He was unable to stay long enough for intravenous infusions so I sent him home with oral supplements and injectable vials of thymus peptides.

Julian returned to my office monthly for three months, during which time the submandibular mass shrank by about half. No new masses were found and all other aspects of his health seemed normal.

He was then, as now, an "active senior," engaging in vigorous outdoor activity including hunting, fishing and hiking as much as eight miles a day.

Over several years his visits to my office were less and less frequent, and by June 28, 1988, his neck was free of palpable masses and he continued to have a normal immune system as measured by live blood analysis. He diligently continued his at-home program, including once-weekly injections, and visited the office once a year.

In May, 1993, he developed pain in the right sacroiliac joint area, buttock, groin and back of the right leg. This was first attributed to a sprain with sciatica since the onset of pain followed heavy lifting.

But on June 9 a bone scan showed an abnormal area in the right sacroiliac joint and an MRI indicated an infiltrative process in the sacral bone involving the upper part and right side of the sacrum with encroachment noted on at least one sacral nerve root.

A biopsy of this area was described as "malignant lymphoma, diffuse, large-cell type." His original microscopic diagnosis had been described as "small-cell type lymphoma."

On July 27, surgery was carried out, removing all accessible cancer from the sacral bone and freeing up the sacral nerve which had been compressed by tumor and which had been causing the severe leg pain. The surgeon had made it clear to the patient and his wife that this operation was for palliation (pain relief) only and that long-term cure was not to be expected. Following the surgery Julian had almost immediate and complete relief of the leg pain and significant relief of back pain.

By August 16, when he visited my office again, he was again able to walk two miles per day with minimal discomfort. While no swollen lymph nodes or other abnormalities were found and his immune function appeared to be adequate, I decided to accelerate the supportive therapy, with more frequent injections and increased dosages of some supplements, particularly vitamin C.

When I saw him again September 13 he had experienced some increased pain in the sacral area, had sleep disturbances primarily due to the pain and noted he was tiring more easily, had become unsteady on arising and was unable to walk as far as usual.

But he also reported to me that over several months prior to the discovery of the continued malignant process he had been suffering from an unusual degree of emotional stress and anxiety. Most of this was internal and had to do with childhood conflicts as well as current relationships.

Typical of most cancer patients, this gentleman had always had some difficulty in verbalizing his deep-rooted and unresolved conflicts. While I had discussed such aspects with him this time I referred him to a professional psychologist in his home area.

On his next visit to my office, October 18, he reported that the counseling had been of great help. Examination on this visit again revealed no findings. However, he still had some tingling sensations in the right sacral area. His oncologist and orthopedist had recommended radiation and heavy chemotherapy upon finding this continued malignancy, and I had backed up the suggestion. But Julian had continued to defer conventional treatment despite his being told such treatment was necessary for his survival.

By November 22, his pain had decreased significantly, his surgical scar had been injected with lidocaine and, even though he felt better and was virtually without pain his home oncologist again suggested radiation. He again declined — but stayed on the immune-supportive program of diet, supplements and weekly thymic peptide injections.

From February 9, 1994, when he felt better than ever and admittedly was "eating like a horse," to the present time, he has physically been in excellent shape. His only negatives have been occasional bouts of emotional distress, which psychological counseling has helped.

The experimental AMAS (Anti-Malignant Antibody in Serum) blood test has been "normal" (that is, not reactive for cancer), darkfield microscopy has indicated constant improvements in immune activity as indicated by white cell activity and aggressiveness, and he has returned to vigorous outdoor activity and hikes nearly 10 miles a day. He has continued to receive weekly thymus injections and to follow the supplementation program. And he has reached age 77 in impressively good shape.

DISCUSSION: Julian has done extremely well with his lymphoma for 10 years. This is despite — or possibly because of — his avoidance of standard treatments of chemotherapy and radiation, even when I supported the idea of the latter. I should point out that both these modalities have frequently been effective in bringing about lengthy remissions in lymphomas and most of us on the "metabolic" side agree they are often necessary in this version of the malignant process.

The only actual "orthodox" modality he followed was pain-relieving, palliative surgery in the sacral area. This was never advocated as, or expected to be, curative.

The second neck node disappeared while on our program and has not reappeared over the past eight years. These observations tend to substantiate my view that such non-toxic, immune-supportive treatments are of benefit with or without orthodox treatment. I emphasize that in their utilization we are not replacing conventional care, but in fact are complementing and enhancing it.

14-YEAR TRIUMPH OVER METASTATIC DENOCARCINOMA

Housewife Diane Baetge, then 40, was still feeling well in April 1982, when she noticed the presence of dark, Burgundy-colored blood in her stool.

Concerned, she consulted her health-maintenance organization (HMO) doctors who ordered an X-ray study of the colon called an air-contrast barium enema, plus the uncomfortable colon probe called a sigmoidoscopy. These tests surprised both her and her doctors by being normal. But the bleeding continued.

In June she underwent a colonoscopy, but the examiner was able to visualize through this technique only up to approximately the lower half of the colon. Nothing was found — but bleeding continued throughout the summer and fall of 1982.

On October 14, after passing a large amount of red blood, she went in for a repeat colonoscopy. This one revealed a large, ulcerating tumor mass in the cecum, the entrance to the large intestine. A biopsy revealed adenocarcinoma, a cancer which often begins in the lower gastrointestinal tract.

On October 21 Diane underwent the surgical removal of the right half of the colon during which time it was determined that cancer had penetrated through the outer wall of the colon into the nearby "pericolic" fat, with "massive involvement of two regional lymph nodes" also noted. The liver was found to be grossly abnormal with obvious metastatic disease. Biopsies of all the involved tissues confirmed metastatic adenocarcinoma as did a lymph node next to the pancreas, thought to be "unresectable" (unremovable) by the surgeon.

As is typical in metastatic colon cancer — whose five-year survival levels under "orthodoxy" have not changed meaningfully in decades — the extensive surgery was followed by chemotherapy in the form of Mitomycin and 5-FU.

The patient herself discontinued the latter because of severe side effects from the chemicals: vomiting, malaise, loss of appetite and loss of hair. She was repeatedly told by her oncologist that if she did not continue her chemotherapy she would "shorten her life." She had also been told by the surgeon following her operation that she had only three to six months to live anyway and that she should "get her affairs in order."

By mid-December 1982, Diane reached the logical conclusion: what was to be lost by seeking an "alternative" form of care?

She came to my facility on Dec. 21, 1982, and began the immune-supportive program of thymus peptides, intravenous vitamins, minerals, laetrile and other nutrients.

At the time of her initial examination in my office, she was found to have several small but definitely enlarged lymph nodes in her neck, along with tenderness just beneath the right rib margin.

After two weeks of vigorous immune support, the discomfort and tenderness previously felt beneath the right rib margin had disappeared and her appetite improved, as did her feeling of well-being.

She then returned home on oral supplements, including enzymes, vitamins, minerals and thymus peptides, along with our cancer prevention diet.

She returned to my facility approximately once per week for two months, on each visit showing improvement in general well-being as well as improvement in immune function as monitored by darkfield microscopy.

CT scans of the abdomen did not reveal any liver lesions, even though there had been at least three palpable masses in the right lobe of the liver at the time of surgery, one of which was biopsied and was positive for metastatic cancer. Scans also failed to reveal any of the cancerous nodes found during the operation, including the inoperable one next to the pancreas.

The patient was then followed in my office at intervals of every two to four months with negative findings until July, 1984, when she developed pain in the right lower chest.

She was found to have localized tenderness over the right front lower rib cage. X-rays of the chest were negative, as was a liver scan, but a bone scan showed a definite abnormality in the sixth rib on the right side corresponding to the area of pain and tenderness and indicating metastatic disease.

Her HMO physicians recommended radiation of the affected area, but the patient declined to have this treatment. Her immune enhancement program was intensified since she had become somewhat less strict with her diet and supplements. Regular injections of the thymus peptides were resumed.

She had also had an increase in stress over the preceding few months and was counseled regarding her manner of coping with it. Over the next six months she experienced a gradual decrease in the chest pain, and on Jan. 22, 1985, a bone scan showed almost complete clearing of the "hot spot" in the right sixth rib. A repeat bone scan in late September, 1985, showed complete resolution of the cancerous activity in the rib. During this interval it was also noted that the mildly enlarged lymph nodes in the neck were no longer detectable.

For the next four years, Diane did very well, with virtually no symptoms or findings until January 1989, when cancer spread to the right fourth and fifth ribs. These were discovered during a bone scan, and were in a different area from the previous involvement. She had had some pain in this area intermittently for several months.

Again her program was intensified and again her symptoms improved.

By December 1989, she was feeling extremely well, exercising, running three miles per day and experiencing only rare episodes of mild pain in the right lower rib cage which would improve with extra doses of the thymus peptides.

By her choice, she was having far less frequent followup visits, both to my clinic and to her HMO doctors. Her last visit to my office was on Sept. 9, 1993, at which time she was doing very well, having only occasional pain in the rib area which was not severe.

During all this time she had rejected radiation therapy, relying solely on non-toxic and non-invasive methods in providing support of her immune system. Because the patient and her husband had moved following this last visit, she was lost to our followup until March 25, 1996, when contact was established through another patient. She was found to be alive and well, continuing with her program.

DISCUSSION: This case demonstrates that the two general modalities, conventional and unconventional, can work together in the best interests of the patient. Having had extensive metastases at the time of her original surgery in 1982 was certainly not in her favor prognostically, at least from the conventional point of view. While I cannot take all of the credit for her remarkable reversal of metastatic disease, since she did have chemotherapy following surgery, I believe that the concomitant use of immune support was a contributing factor in this success story.

The reversal of the metastatic disease in the rib in 1984, and again in 1989, occurred without standard radiation therapy, so I feel that some credit must be given to her use of alternative methods. The conventional view of bony metastases is that they do not come and go, and that they do not disappear without radiation or some conventional treatment. This case would tend to refute this concept. As with other cases I have seen, the long survival of 14 years after discovery of metastases is remarkable in itself.

And even more important is the nagging question: what would have happened if this patient, sensing something wrong in April 1982, had gone on an anti-cancer dietary program with supplements and had not waited six months before her cancer was diagnosed?

KEEPING HER BREAST — OR MOST OF IT

Pat Smith, then 49, was aware of the growing plague of breast cancer in the Western world, with an incidence level reaching, as of 1996, either 1 out of 9 women or 1 out of 8, depending on who's counting.

In mid-April 1992, Mrs. Smith, a switchboard operator and housewife, first noticed the dreaded lump in her left breast. A month later a "suspicious" mammogram and a needle-guided excisional biopsy confirmed a variety of malignancy called "infiltrating ductal and intraductal carcinoma." Pathology also indicated that some cancer remained in her breast.

Conventional thinking, as expressed by her surgeon, was that she needed a radical mastectomy — complete removal of the breast and surrounding lymph nodes — a challenge faced by hundreds of thousands of American women annually.

Mrs. Smith pleaded with her surgeon to do a simple lumpectomy — removal of the immediate cancerous tissue — to be able to spare her breast. He steadfastly refused.

Aware that alternatives existed, she sought out my practice. She was not trying to avoid conventional care, but she was of the belief she could be "built up" to undergo whatever surgery or other treatment might be required. And she was aware that since her mother and a cousin had died of breast cancer at a young age and her own biopsy had shown a high degree of malignancy, her prognosis was guarded at best.

I found a 2 cm. X 3 cm. mass and, by darkfield microscopy, a low level of immune performance in an otherwise healthy woman.

She immediately went on my immune augmentation program with daily intravenous infusions of vitamins, (particularly of C), minerals (including selenium, germanium, magnesium, potassium) and laetrile. These IV "drips," along with intramuscular injections of thymus peptides, went on for three weeks.

I next placed her on oral supplements including vitamins A and E, proteolytic enzymes, and oral glandulars (thymus, adrenal, lymph, lymph tissues, bone marrow), all designed to improve immune function.

Over her initial three-week period her immune function, measured by white blood cell activity, improved from about 20 percent to 100 percent of normal.

The patient then returned home on an oral program and special diet. She remained in contact with her surgeon, repeatedly asking if he would consider less than a full mastectomy.

Finally he relented and opted for removal of a fourth or quadrant of the whole breast encompassing the area of the remaining tumor.

A few weeks later I received a telephone call from Patricia, who told me elatedly that the tissue that had been removed contained no cancer. A pathologist report confirming this was later sent to me.

About 2½ months later the experimental AMAS blood test was "normal."

The patient returned for a followup visit in March 1995, some eight months after her surgery. She had been under an unusual amount of stress over the preceding weeks, and had been feeling progressively more tired over the month or so prior to her visit. She had also been having headaches, which were unusual for her.

Upon her return visit the examination of her breast failed to reveal any masses, nor were there any other positive physical findings. However, the darkfield microscope showed a drop in viability and activity of the white blood cells, indicating a decrease in the ability of her immune system to cope with disease.

I decided to attempt to restore her immune system with IV supplementation similar to that which had been administered initially. This was carried out over a week's time, and was followed by a satisfactory improvement in white blood cell activity. The patient was also counseled about the importance of stress reduction, and I went into considerable detail as to the specific stress factors which appeared to be affecting her adversely. I re-emphasized to her that if these obstacles were not overcome or dealt with as positively as possible, she might very well experience a recurrence of her disease.

A followup visit occurred in October 1995, by which time she had made several adjustments in her living situation with the help of a supportive husband. Her mood was greatly improved, as were her energy level and feeling of well-being. Her immune function was vastly improved over that of the first day of the previous visit.

In a telephone call on March 19, 1996, I found her to be in an excellent state of mind and health. She had just had a checkup by her local oncologist who had found no lumps in the breasts or other abnormalities on physical examination. Her cancer "markers" were normal, as was a mammogram.

DISCUSSION: Despite the short term, this case is a graphic description of how so-called "orthodox" and "alternative" therapies can work together and how the traumatizing radical mastectomy, which may do as much damage to a woman's self-esteem as to the body itself, can often be avoided. It also demonstrates how important the mind and attitudes are in helping the patient hold the line against the malignant process — which, again, is never "cured" but may be amenable to long-term control.

A 17-YEAR CONTROL OF MALIGNANT LYMPHOMA

The case of 35-year-old Kay Harper began in June 1979 when a diagnosis by biopsy of an enlarged lymph gland in the neck was lymphoma.

But from the first moment she opted for "alternative" or immune-supportive therapy, and found her way to the Richardson Clinic in Albany, California, where I was filling in for Dr. Richardson on a part-time basis.

Some of the records of this patient's impressive case are no longer available, but there are enough of them for a reasonably accurate account to be assembled.

In July 1979 Kay developed "ascites," or fluid accumulation, in the abdomen. I performed a paracentesis, or draining of the fluid, on July 19, which yielded about five quarts of fluid containing malignant cells.

I then carried out several "taps" and injected the protein-digesting enzyme complex Wobe-Mugos into the abdominal cavity.

In August, she developed progressive shortness of breath, and on August 14 she was found to have fluid in both chest cavities, or pleural spaces (outside the lungs), with more fluid present in the left side.

The left chest was tapped and drained, yielding about two quarts of amber fluid. This was followed by the injection of the enzyme material.

About a week later, another thoracentesis, or draining of the left chest cavity, was carried out and again the enzyme mixture was introduced into the pleural space. On each occasion the patient felt better and was able to breathe more easily after the procedure.

Over the next several months the left pleural space was tapped several times, with decreasing amounts of fluid recovered each time, and with the enzymes injected on each occasion.

On April 20, 1980, she was admitted to a Reno hospital by a local oncologist because of persistent swelling of the abdomen. CT scans showed enlargement of the liver and spleen as well as a large abdominal mass, or more likely a confluent string of masses probably representing enlarged retroperitoneal lymph nodes, presumably malignant.

Scans also showed the persistence of fluid in the abdominal cavity as well as some recurrence of fluid, or pleural effusions, in both chest cavities. Biopsy of a lymph node under the left arm was done on April 21, 1980, and this was first interpreted as malignant histiocytosis by pathologists at Stanford University.

Specimens were also sent to pathologists at the University of Southern California, who disagreed and called it metastatic carcinoma or metastatic sarcoma.

In spite of the uncertainty in diagnosis, the patient was treated with chemotherapy, consisting of Cytoxan, Oncovin, Adriamycin and Prednisone. She had prompt and dramatic relief of her abdominal distention and shortness of breath, with reduction of the abdominal fluid and resolution of the pleural effusions.

This chemotherapy regimen had been previously enhanced in my office with IV vitamins and minerals as well as DMSO.

She was discharged from the hospital on April 29, 1980, in a much improved condition and with virtually no symptoms. She was instructed by the oncologist in Reno to continue the chemotherapy with the oncologist in her home area in Colorado, but she chose not to do so. She then did well until October 1980, when she began to develop headaches along with intermittent episodes of numbness in her right hand and right upper lip.

She returned to Reno where a consultation was held with a highly competent neurologist who carried out a brain scan, EEG, or brain wave test, and a complete neurological examination. He was unable to find any explanation for her symptoms.

The symptoms progressed to the point where she developed a stiff neck, fever, blindness, extreme lethargy, finally becoming stuporous and intermittently in a coma, unable to respond to questions or to stimuli. She was obviously acutely and severely ill. She was again referred to the Reno oncologist, who carried out further testing, including a spinal tap, which revealed malignant cells in the spinal fluid.

On October 11, 1980, a chemotherapeutic drug, Methotrexate, was injected into the spinal canal. Following this, because of the finding of malignancy in her brain, a stent or small catheter was placed into the affected area of the brain to facilitate the direct injection of Methotrexate, which was done weekly for five weeks.

Her speech returned and headache disappeared after the first treatment. Vision gradually improved over the next two months, but with intermittent recurrences of blind spots in her central vision, which eventually disappeared. Radiation of the brain was also carried out from October 15 through October 28, 1980.

Throughout all of this conventional treatment, Kay was continuing with her immune support program, including vitamins A,E,C, antioxidants, etc., including some injections of polypeptides. She tolerated all treatments very well, with minimal nausea following one or two of the chemotherapeutic injections.

The numbness of the lip and hand disappeared after the first or second injection and never returned.

She was seen and examined in my office annually over the next few years, and on each occasion was found to be free of swelling, fluid, lymph node enlargement, neurological or any other physical findings. Blood counts, chemistries, and cancer markers remained negative.

Her last examination in my office was on July 2, 1985, but subsequent phone contacts have revealed that this lady, now 52, remains alive and well (the last contact was March 20, 1996). Distance and her busy schedule do not permit regular visits to Reno, but checkups in her home area have failed to reveal any recurrence of her cancer. She has faithfully continued on her supplement program, diet, stress reduction, and a generally healthy lifestyle.

DISCUSSION: This case demonstrates that there are some patient conditions and situations in which conventional chemotherapy and other traditional methods must be relied upon. The oncologists, of course, claim the victory in this case, and I believe rightly so, to a great extent. However, judging from this as well as other cases, I believe the concomitant use of immune-enhancing substances can be complementary, and at the very least can minimize the adverse effects of chemotherapy and radiation.

It should also be pointed out that it is unusual to see such a long survival time (17 years) following metastatic cancer involving liver, abdominal cavity, lymph nodes, chest cavity, and brain, with the additional possibility — by orthodox reasoning — of different "types" of cancer, particularly in view of the fact that the patient received only a fraction of the standard course or dosage of the chemotherapeutic drugs.

Regarding the interesting possibility of her having two different "types" of cancer, those of us who approach cancer as a deficiency disease tend to feel that cancer is cancer and that the fine distinctions made by pathologists are less important than what we view as the basic problem of a breakdown of immune function. We should view this case as a victory for the combined efforts of conventional and alternative methodologies.

BEATING PROSTATE CANCER 'UNCONVENTIONALLY'

In December, 1989, Phil Canville, then age 62, was seen at Kaiser Hospital, Walnut Creek, California, for passing stones in the urine thought to be from the prostate. He then underwent studies of the prostate, including biopsies, which were considered to be benign.

In August 1990, the patient was admitted to Kaiser with severe pain in the right side of his abdomen and back, having had this intermittently over the previous six weeks. He was found to have a kidney stone which passed spontaneously with the aid of medication.

On this occasion, a nodule or lump was discovered in Phil's prostate gland, which was confirmed by sonogram. This prostate module was not directly related to the kidney stone or to the symptoms which brought him to the hospital, but was found coincidentally in the course of the initial examination. Biopsy of this mass revealed it to be malignant. There was microscopic evidence of cancerous invasion of the perineural (around nerves) lymphatics (lymph channels) within the prostate.

A CT scan of the pelvis showed no evidence of involvement of pelvic lymph nodes or other pelvic structures. However, a bone scan revealed two small areas in the left scapula (shoulder blade), suspicious for metastatic disease. Phil was told by his Kaiser urologist in no uncertain terms that he must have either surgery — namely, radical prostatectomy — or radiation, and that he must decide which of these modalities he would accept within 30 days or face dire consequences.

After carefully considering all of his treatment options, and spending considerable time investigating alternative modalities, Phil elected to pursue the latter and came to my office, then in Incline Village, in mid-September 1990. There a review of his Kaiser records, a complete history and physical examination were done. The latter confirmed the presence of a small nodule in the left lobe of the prostate.

I placed him on an immune-enhancing program consisting of proper diet, enzymes, vitamins and supplements as discussed elsewhere (*see Chapter VI*). This was followed in a few days by intravenous infusions of high-dose vitamins, including vitamin C, B-complex, folic acid, and B-17 (laetrile), along with minerals such as zinc, germanium, selenium, magnesium and potassium.   Intramuscular injections of thymus extract and thymus peptides were also given. I continued this program for five weeks, along with the IV infusions. Phil was also started on Flutamide, a conventional medication which interferes with the influence of male hormones on the prostate and thus on prostate cancer.

This medicine had to be stopped after a month because of severe tenderness of the nipples, a common side effect of male hormone blockers. Later, he took Flutamide in a reduced dosage — one or two capsules per day, as compared to the usual six capsules daily. Along with this program, he was given injections of an autologous vaccine (made from the patient's own blood serum) for additional immune enhancement.

It is interesting to note that this patient's PSA (Prostate Specific Antigen) never became elevated, this being unusual in cases of proven cancer of the prostate.

Over the next several years, Phil visited my office on a regular basis — at first monthly, then every two or three months — on each occasion having an evaluation of his immune system by means of live cell analysis, along with other testing. In some visits, when his health and immune function were considered to be less than optimal, he would be given an immune "boost" with several IV infusions similar to those administered over the first three weeks. This was not required often, because this man, to me, was the ideal patient, who was faithfully taking his supplements, following his diet, and making the necessary changes in his lifestyle to bring about the desired result.

Phil's last visit to my office, now in Reno, Nevada, was on July 31, 1995, at which time he was found to be in excellent general health. The PSA was normal at 2.3. Sonograms of the prostate showed no change, and there had been basically no change in this "picture" of the prostate over the previous five years; if anything, the tumor appeared to be possibly a little smaller.

His immune function remained excellent, as it had for the most part throughout the duration of his care.

On September 10, 1996, a phone conversation with Phil revealed that a sonogram done by Kaiser showed no evidence of tumor!   Copies of the sonogram have been received and reviewed, confirming this.

DISCUSSION: The remarkable aspect of this case is that Phil Canville received no conventional therapy other than the anti-male hormone medication, which had to be taken only intermittently and in reduced dosage because of his apparent difficulty in tolerating it.   In spite of his refusal to have the "life-saving" radical prostatectomy, Phil has not only survived for six years with an excellent quality of life, but has apparently beaten the odds even further by seeing his tumor disappear.

Time, of course, will tell as to how lasting this apparent remission will be, but my view is that Phil's future looks much brighter than it would have had he limited himself to conventional treatment alone.

Chapter III
THE CANCER CATASTROPHE
Losing the Deadly War

"Morale is sagging."

This is the way the *Congressional Quarterly* in 1996 described both the cancer situation in the United States and the National Cancer Institute (NCI), the federally funded research conduit which sits at the scientific apex of what many call the Cancer Establishment or Cancer Inc.

The legislative publication was assessing the first quarter-century since President Richard M. Nixon had declared the "War on Cancer" — actually the Conquest of Cancer program — in 1971.

As of 1996, yet another new skipper at the NCI, Dr. Richard Klausner, was aboard to offer equal doses of optimism and concern.

His predecessor, Dr. Samuel Broder, who, as is common with government bigwigs, had left the NCI to join private industry, had begun *his* five-year reign with almost bubbly enthusiasm about progress being made against the nation's number-two "natural" killer.

Yet, several things had become apparent during the Broder period:

— Despite billions of dollars dumped into the Conquest of Cancer program, there was more cancer among more sectors of the population at ever earlier ages than ever before.

— Cancer rates were climbing higher than ever before with each passing year.

— The combined direct/indirect cost of treating this rapidly growing malady was calculated, as of the mid-1990s, to be at least $200 *billion* a year.

Yet there was one ray of hope on the horizon:

For the first time, the US cancer mortality rate actually showed a decrease — 2.6% between 1991 and 1995, as contrasted with an increase of 6.4% between 1971 and 1990. Most of the decline was due to a decrease in cigarette smoking and earlier diagnostics — that is, it had little to do with successes of actual treatments.

The *incidence* of cancer, however, has continued to climb, (by a startling 18.6% for men and 12.4% for women between 1978-1991), which offsets enthusiasm for a slight decrease in cancer fatalities.

Some statistical manipulations on the one hand seem to bolster Cancer Inc.'s notion that people are living longer with cancer, yet they also confirm that more cancer is occurring.

Using already outdated numbers, some of these based on 1991-1993, the Cancer Establishment was 'fessing up to about 600,000 deaths per year — even though overviews of data extrapolated in 1995 made it fairly clear that the truer figure was at least 700,000 deaths per year. The American Cancer Society (ACS) incidence data showed a staggering 1.9 million new cases being diagnosed that year.

One author (Culbert), assessing both the "solid" data from immediate years past and "projected" or estimated figures, found that, in terms of the clock, by the end of this decade cancer may be killing one American approximately every 45 seconds, or as many as 1900 per day, the same 24-hour period in which some 5,200 new cases will be diagnosed.

All figures are awesomely higher than in 1971, when President Richard Nixon had announced an all-out war on cancer under the naive belief that if enough money could be raised and tagged for research into "the Big C" that surely the disease could at last be cured. His political associates, some affiliated with Cancer Inc., had said so, and he obviously believed so. It would not be the first time a political leader had been so misled by a scientific establishment held hostage to vested interests.

By 1996, there were various ways to describe what the facts really meant:

One out of three Americans now living is — statistically — doomed to get cancer.

One of every five Americans now living is — statistically — doomed to die of the disease.

It now affects two out of three families to one degree or another.

It is now the biggest "natural" — that is, non-accidental, non-homicidal, non-suicidal — killer of the very young and among the top killers of the middle-aged and very old. It is growing among "minorities" even at a faster clip than among Caucasians.

And, there is a sobering adjunctive reality:

The increase in cancer is general throughout the entire *Western* world, although there are some national and regional variations.

What this means, for example, is that Western nations with populations smaller than the USA (265 million) are more immediately threatened, literally with extinction, than is the USA. Among such "sentinel" countries are Iceland (270,000) and New Zealand (3.5 million), literally poles apart but both bearing similar increasing rates of cancer (and other metabolic, chronic and immunological disorders).

And, in terms of near-time forecasting, things don't get much better:

Chances are that by the turn of the millenium cancer will be affecting 1 out of every 2 Americans (and, probably, citizens of the Western world) and that oncology will be the number-one medical specialty going into the 21st century, bypassing cardiology.

Yet even so, year by year — often just as the Cancer Society gets ready for yet another fund drive — Cancer Inc. has beguiled the American population with stories of the "great breakthroughs" that lie "at the end of the tunnel" as we "turn the corner" on cancer. It seems that just another couple of billions will do the job -- rhetoric we heard so often when deployed during the Vietnam War.

As recently as 1990, the nation's top cancer experts were crowing over "the fact" that "at least half of cancer is curable" — again, understanding cure to mean five years free of symptoms. The optimism came because, for the first time, five-year survivals had just barely crossed the 50% threshold.

But as dissidents were quick to note, there was a lot of numbers juggling in all this: first, the real net gain in American oncology has been in improved diagnostics. This means that cancer may be detected earlier than it was decades ago. Earlier detection does not mean cancer therapies work any better, only that the time from detection to death has lengthened.

And, second, five-year survivals of non-melanoma skin cancers, localized cancers of the cervix, and some other non-spreading (metastasizing) cancers detected early in specific sites, have been "curable" (that is, amenable to five-year absences of symptoms) since the days of Ptolemy. By including the simple cancers, such as skin cancers and early cancer of the cervix, with the killers and winding the survival clock back a notch to account for earlier diagnostics some apparent "progress" in the "war on cancer" can be seen.

But it fades as the harsh realities become clear and it is manifest that the number of the "killer cancers" — metastatic cancer spread from one site to vital organs — are worse in terms of incidence and mortality than ever before despite all the vaunted "breakthroughs" annually announced.

It has taken the general population, threatened in ever greater numbers in each succeeding decade, seemingly a very long time to get the central message. But it is coming through — and, as the movement for "alternative medicine" now so clearly shows — it is coming through loud and clear.

Most of what American medical orthodoxy knows, thinks or does about cancer has mostly been wrong most of the time. Never before in medical history has so much treasure been squandered in such vast numbers on so many ideas that are basically defective.

And never before have such extensive sectors of the public begun to question the revealed wisdom of the medical establishment as they are now doing concerning cancer.

Given the above statistics, it is not difficult to see why a majority of Americans have long equated the word "cancer" with "death" — and why so many, first by the hundreds, then by the thousands, then by the scores of thousands, fled American cancer orthodoxy when they could, either seeking out "alternative" practitioners like myself or heading for Mexico or anywhere else where they might have a better chance to save their lives.

It simply rubs the everyday American the wrong way:

Just how can the world's most technologically advanced, and certainly most expensive, medical system be such an utter failure with such an awful disease, particularly when there has been such an enormous public-private effort to understand and stop it?

How can the American space program, with some notable exceptions, log one spectacular victory after another as mankind blasts into the cosmos and plans for landings on other worlds (as his expertly manufactured spacecraft plunge into deep space billions of miles away on journeys whose final stop cannot even be contemplated by ordinary minds) yet cancer remains unsolved on Planet Earth?

Given the grim cancer reality — and the federal research expense alone of $25 billion in the first quarter-century of the "war on cancer" — why *shouldn't* an advanced cancer patient cast a wary eye on current methodology?

After all, however worse the cancer rates, and however many billions of dollars have been spent on cancer research, the orthodox approach to cancer — with the exception of adding immunotherapy as a "fourth leg" — has hardly varied over the years.

The approach is meted out through what we call Cancer Inc:

The highly propagandistic and private American Cancer Society (ACS), the governmental coordinating National Cancer Institute (NCI), and a spiderweb of public-private-academic research laboratories and spinoff industries in surgery, toxic chemicals, radiation, artificial hormones, genetically engineered "immune-boosting" proteins, ever-changing blood tests, cancer markers, monitoring and detecting devices and other elements of high-tech diagnostics.

Its focus remains on the malignant tumor, or tumors, and how to cut, burn, poison or otherwise eradicate them from the body in the 17th-century belief that cancer *is* tumors and that the absence of tumors somehow equates with the absence of cancer.

Numerous exposés have indicated just how this faulty logic has helped prop up the numerous interconnected cancer industries. Even so, at mid-decade, oncology (from root words really meaning "the study of bumps") is essentially vested in these therapeutic approaches:

SURGERY: the idea that removing malignant tissue, and often nearby ostensibly affected tissue and possibly adjacent lymph nodes, will somehow be "removing the cancer."

Advancing from past centuries to the earlier part of the present one, surgery was for generations the *only* treatment for the malignant process. And, truth to tell, because simple surgical removals of accessible tumors often did equate with "five years free of symptoms" (the surgical gold standard which became the essential measurement in oncology's weird definition of the word "cure"), so that a patient might live long enough to die of something else, there was, and there still remains, a valid reason for surgery.

RADIATION: borrowed from the ancients (who believed tumors could be burned off by fire) and stimulated by Curie, Grubbe *et al.,* this approach seeks to burn out or off a tumor. Cobalt and other items may be used in the "radiating" of a tumor area, an internal blowtorch approach which, unfortunately, often does as much damage to normal as malignant tissues while lowering patient host defense (immunity). But, again, because an affected mass may be reduced for a certain length of time, there was, and is, some justification for the limited use of radiation, particularly against fast-growing tumors not apt to be stopped by any other method.

CHEMOTHERAPY: perhaps the most controversial (and industrially profitable) of the methods, in this approach toxic chemicals which either directly attack cancer cells or interfere with their ability to "replicate" are used against cancer body-wide. Unfortunately, such chemicals poison not only cancer cells but normal ones as well, giving rise to the need for drugs to counter the side effects of the cancer drugs or to "rescue" patients from their overdoses. The side effects of toxic anti-cancer compounds range from gastrointestinal disturbances (vomiting, acute diarrhea, spasms) to hair loss, skin lesions, immunological weakening, liver and kidney damage, bone marrow depression and a long list of other hideous sequelae. Year by year, new "experimental" cancer drugs, alone or in combination, have been hawked as possible "cures" for this or that "form" of cancer, usually meaning the possibility of attaining the golden five years without symptoms and equating the same as "cures." And, in some simpler, non-spreading "forms" of the disease, chemotherapy seems truly to have effected just such a "cure."

In recent years, and owing in no small extent to some of the ideas being advanced by metabolic and holistic doctors (often derided as "quacks" at an earlier time), orthodox oncology has added its "fourth leg" to the Traditional Triad:

IMMUNOTHERAPY. Yet orthodoxy does not exactly mean by "immuno-therapy" what some of us do. Metabolic doctors have long said (and, as we shall see, the biochemical evidence now strongly indicates) that many natural elements, particularly in nutrition, can be used to enhance or modulate a damaged immune system and that such enhancement or modulation is the key to disease prevention. Such doctors also believe that immunity might be better described as "host defense," since not all aspects of such a system are well understood and classical immunology often refers to several sets of immune system cells whose functions are fairly well understood.

Orthodoxy has concentrated on manufactured, and often genetically engineered, artificial proteins, particularly "interferons" (mimicking the activity of natural anti-infective, anticancer agents in the body) and "interleukins" (working as synthetic hormones) in efforts to "jack up" parts of a lagging immune system as the latter may relate to cancer. The trouble with such products has been that they are (a) often highly toxic in dosages used conventionally, (b) extremely expensive, and (c) at least so far, mostly ineffective.

For some time, orthodox oncology pinned its highest of hopes on the artificial new proteins which would somehow obliterate tumors by marshalling an immune response against them. To many of us, this was the perversion of a good idea: vitamins, minerals, enzymes, amino acids, and essential fatty acids may indeed help the immune system, at a far less expensive, far more effective and far less dangerous level. But the same have largely been "outside the paradigm" and certainly outside of the cancer industry.

There is now developing, as we will also see later, a "fifth leg":

GENETICS: This is a natural outgrowth of the idea that mutated genes are the "cause" of cancer and that new genetic weapons may be designed to correct such mutations or to head off their damage or to stimulate responses against them. There is much excitement about all this in the 1990s — just as there was about viruses and cancer in the 1970s. I may be an outsider, but I hope and pray — and in fact assume — that something of benefit will come out of the genetic approach. One would think that if so much money is being spent on so many projects at least some of them should pan out.

As to the Traditional Triad — surgery, radiation and chemotherapy — it has become obvious over the decades that while all three may impact on a cancer patient's immunity (so that even if many cancer cells have been killed he may die of a simple bacterial infection he cannot fight off naturally), the latter two are often associated with "secondary cancer" later!

This does not mean, as we stress again and again, that there are not times and places for any or *all* of these modalities. In an integrative model, as I champion, anything that works constitutes preferred treatment. And, as I note elsewhere (*see VII*), it is now clear that certain elements of nutritional or metabolic therapy, particularly the antioxidants, actually enhance the healing powers of chemotherapy and radiation.

Such incredible realities were among reasons why I turned toward more natural forms of healing — not only in cancer, but medicine in general.

I am more than ever convinced from my experience that many of the "alternative" methods of healing are successful where orthodox methods are not.

The basic difference between the two approaches is more philosophical than technical. We of the unorthodox persuasion believe that cancer is basically a deficiency or breakdown of the defense system, while orthodoxy views cancer as a foreign invader which must be destroyed at all costs. To us, the costs — in terms of suffering, secondary cancers, and even death directly attributed to treatment — are too often prohibitive.

Chapter IV
MALIGNANCY AND METABOLIC MAYHEM
Theories on the Nature of Cancer

There is not a cancer-treating doctor out there who does not know that at least to some degree he or she is firing in the dark — simply because nobody yet fully understands the nature of the beast, a key reason why so much orthodox cancer therapy fails.

The word itself is derived from the Latin word for crab, *cancrum*, because so much surface cancer (sarcoma, we suspect) seemed in ancient times to spread over the body in a disjointed form closer in appearance to a crab than anything else.

It is conventional wisdom that there may have been a lot more cancer around in antiquity than we are aware of, and that a lot of disease conditions may have been manifestations of what medicine today calls cancer. The same observation holds for the presence of cancer in more primitive societies today.

Even so, the conclusion is inescapable that — however we are defining the term — cancer is far more prominent among the supposedly "civilized" peoples and in the modern era than it is among the less-civilized ones and among people who lived in past eras. It is, simply put, more than anything a disease of civilization — something civilization is doing to itself.

After all, for years, hardly a week has gone by without the announcement that this or that chemical, food, gas, emission, activity or behavior has been identified as a "cause" of a "kind" of cancer. For all intents and purposes, according to orthodox thought, almost everything "causes" cancer — at least in the Western world.

What the orthodox medical establishment seems to have difficulty comprehending is that cancer as a process is not foreign to the human body — since each of us produces hundreds of thousands of cancer cells every day! This simple fact hence makes it ludicrous to attempt a therapy which is aimed at destroying every last cancer cell in the body.

The way in which the body handles these aberrant cells — that is, the overall host defense system including all aspects of immunity — determines whether or not such cell proliferation, a subclinical malignant process, actually results in clinical (diagnosable, detectable) cancer.

Oncological experts generally agree that cancer is a process in which a cell, for some reason, remains immature and "undifferentiated" and results in uncontrolled growth. The process is often characterized by rapid spread ("metastasis") and invasion of both local and distant tissues. Visually, the process is more often than not defined as a "tumor type" or a mass of cells clustered as a space-occupying new growth ("neoplasm") susceptible to change in shape, color, size and the ability to spread to other sites.

Our modern-era, severely compartmentalized medicine has given birth to modern-era, severely particularized oncology ("the study of bumps") which categorizes types of cancer cells and tissues under various names. Depending on who's counting and from what angle, there hence are said to be several hundred "types" or "forms" of cancer. Those related to various solid tissues are broadly classed as carcinomas or sarcomas, those relating to the blood as leukemias, and there are other varieties and mixtures of the above.

Since so much modern or standard (allopathic) medicine is involved in naming, classifying and treating pathological entities rather than treating causes, it is common to speak of a malignant mass in the breast as "breast cancer" (typically a carcinoma), and of a malignant mass in the colon as "colon cancer" (typically an adenocarcinoma), which gives rise to the — in my mind — unfortunate conclusion that there are many separate diseases, each needing its own treatment. This linchpin of oncological thought has given rise to the cancer industry — the churning out of therapies designed primarily to eradicate the signs and symptoms of the malignant process (usually tumor masses, enlarged spleens, excess white cells, as common examples) through the aforementioned trinity of surgery, radiation and chemotherapy, belatedly joined by immunotherapy and genetics-based approaches.

The concept of "curing" cancer has long depended on the assumption that the vanishing of symptoms and signs (most typically, tumor destruction) for five years constitutes just such an outcome. And it is true that the destruction or removal of either slowly-spreading or essentially non-spreading skin lesions or accessible single-site tumors has often led to long periods of survival in which such symptoms did not reappear. These have been considered "cures" of cancer. To others, though, they have been signs that the malignant process itself remained essentially under control, if not cured, so that an individual lived long enough to die of something else.

And, giving the devil his oncological due, there are cases of metastatic cancer — that is, malignant manifestations spread from one site to another — in which standard therapies, in eliminating enough of the symptoms and manifestations without in turn killing the host, have effected a five-year survival rate without symptoms — hence, a "cure."

Many of those of us on the metabolic or holistic side do not believe that the elimination of a symptom or one of the manifestations constitutes the cure of a disease. More likely, the capability of a cancer patient to withstand the devastating attack of surgery, chemotherapy and radiation as it demonstrably reduces some of the cancer load speaks more to the patient's innate powers of self-defense (overall immunity) than to the successes of cancer treatments, for all the standard ones in some way impair, harm, damage or in some way lower the defenses of the patient.

As the decade comes to a close, theories as to the nature and origin of cancer fall into two categories:

POLYPATHOLOGY: the prevalent view that there are some two hundred "forms" or "types" or "subtypes" of cancer, each with a separate cause of cluster of causes and each thus needing a separate variety or combination of varieties of treatments.

UNITARIANISM: the idea that there is a single *malignant process*, whose advance may result in all the features and manifestations confused by the polypathologists as cancer itself.

Therapeutic victory over cancer does not depend on the primacy of either theory. End results are always more important than theory.

It is probably safe to say that, in keeping with our general views on medicine, those of us on the metabolic/holistic side generally have favored unitarianism, if by no means in agreement as to what that unitarian nature may be.

The target of the metabolic or holistic therapist is not simply the removal or diminution of the gross manifestation of cancer (usually a tumor or tumors) but rather the elimination or mitigation of the underlying process which gave rise to them. This is the single major conceptual/therapeutic difference between standard allopaths and metabolically oriented physicians.

This is why so many metabolically oriented cancer-treating doctors, under attack by their medical boards for allegedly "controversial" approaches to cancer, correctly argue that they basically are not treating tumors but indeed the whole body, that they are less interested in managing symptoms than they are in eliminating causes. Such an utterance is, even at this late date, often regarded by the oncological establishment as arrant nonsense.

However, epidemiology and biochemistry are tending more and more to favor the "alternative" position on cancer: that it is largely a product of civilization, that the primary elements of civilization which most affect it are diet (the sum total of eating habits together with the problems wrought by the food-processing industry) along with the stresses and distresses of our modern society, and that initially cancer is probably a unitarian malignant process, whatever its ultimate symptoms and manifestations may be.

Orthodox views of cancer causation have switched dizzyingly in the past few decades, and, with the advent of genetics, they are now tending to dovetail with the unitarian concept.

For most of the last half of this century, the discipline of virology was turned to help "explain" cancer. The idea that cancer is somehow a foreign disease, alien to the body, "caused" by something, is a natural adjunct of allopathic thinking, since the allopathic paradigm (treatment by contraries) presupposes that illness is the result of disease-causing entities — be they bacteria, yeasts, parasites, fungi, mycoplasmas,and later viruses — and hence that ridding oneself of such entities results in health.

For some four decades the virological approach to understanding cancer was dominant, and it was the primary concept when the "War on Cancer" was declared in 1971.

However, after decades of research, it has become impossible to make a specific case for any virus actually causing a human malignancy other than in some "close relationships" — such as HTLV-1's close relationship with a rare disorder called adult T-cell leukemia; human papilloma virus' close relationship with certain epithelial "cancers" (uterine cervix, anogenital area, vulva, etc.); the Epstein-Barr virus' close relationship with several "kinds" of tumors, including immunoblastic lymphoma, Burkitt's lymphoma and possibly Hodgkin's; the close relationship between hepatitis B and C viruses with liver cancer; and, more recently, the close relationship between reputed KSHV (Kaposi's sarcoma-associated human herpesvirus) and the most common "cancer type" in AIDS.

But "close relationship" — or correlation — is not necessarily causation, a point forcefully made by Berkeley molecular biologist Peter Duesberg in his incessant attack on the HIV theory of AIDS causation. **(1)** The presence of DNA or RNA "sequences" and/or viral particles in tumor systems indicates relationship; it does not prove causation.

On Sept. 16, 1995, *The Lancet* published a telling survey which indicated paradigm shift:

J.D.H. Morris *et al.* of Great Britain concluded succinctly:

"Infection with specific viruses has a role in the pathogenesis of some cancers in human beings. However, the incidence of such cancers is much lower than the frequency of virus infection, suggesting that infection alone does not result in cancer and that cellular events in addition to the presence of the virus must occur, or that cancer occurs only if viral proteins are expressed in an inappropriate cell type or in an immunocompromised host." **(2)**

The phrase "immunocompromised host" opens the door widely to the metabolic/holistic perspective: the overall defense system of the host is more important than the offending virus, a restatement of the host-vs.-terrain argument of the French medical school of the 19th century at the time of the advent of the microbial theory of disease.

Morris *et al.* added further:

"It is now clear that acquisition of a malignant phenotype usually requires accumulation of multiple genetic changes by the cell." **(3)**

Hence another door is opened — to the higher-tech world of genetics, which is now beginning to supersede the viral (or any other) orthodox theory as to the nature of cancer.

It has been pointed out by cancer research dissidents that the race of cancer orthodoxy to embrace genes as the "cause" of all cancer was simply a switch within the same research establishment from the embrace of viruses as the "cause" of all cancer as the latter theory failed.

And geneticists themselves have cautioned about going overboard with the genetic theory.

As University of Michigan geneticist Dr. Charles Sing told *Newsweek*:

"What is a good gene and what is a bad gene depend on how you treat it.

"Genes don't wake up until they are exposed to some environmental factor." **(4)**

And, interestingly, it is genetics — the *creme de la creme* of modern research — which is pointing the way to a unitarian thesis, for hardly a month has gone by since the early 1990s without a new gene being discovered whose mutation somehow is said to be involved in "causing" a "kind" of cancer. And now there are genes said to lurk behind multiple "causes" of cancer.

In 1996, Dr. Martson Linehan of the National Cancer Institute (NCI) described the discovery of a gene called FHIT as "the Rosetta stone of cancer study." **(5)** This gene is said to "cause" a vast variety of cancers (esophagus, stomach, colon, respiratory, lung, breast). This was years after delineation of mutated gene p53, thought to be a near-universal cancer "cause," and of a range of genes related to specific cancers.

For years, laetrile advocates also championed the controversial and usually condemned "trophoblastic theory of cancer," advanced at the turn of the century by Scottish embryologist John Beard. This intriguing theory simply stated that the invasive, corrosive trophoblast tissue so necessary to the process of pregnancy and birth shares so many characteristics with cancer tissue that cancer is, more than anything, simply misplaced trophoblast. And that whatever inhibits trophoblast growth — such as pancreatic enzymes — should do the same for cancer. Hence the early advent of enzyme therapy against cancer.

Modern research has strongly indicated that cancer and trophoblast are not identical, but there are properties in both which point to a cancer unitarianism. The primary one is human chorionic gonadotropin (hCG), a hormone found in all cancers as well as cultured embryonic and fetal cells while absent in benign tumors.

Continuing years of research in this area, the Allegheny-Singer Research Institute's Dr. Hernan F. Acevedo and colleagues announced in 1995 that a further study of five fetal "cell lines" and 28 "cancer cell lines," while reconfirming the researchers' earlier findings on hCG ubiquity, also found the genetic links therein — that hCG beta gene activation was occurring in both cancer and fetal cells,

"indicating that at any given time there is the possibility of activation of as many as four genes of the six genes of the

hCG-(beta)-HLB (beta) gene cluster . . . (results which) support the concept that cancer is a problem of development and differentiation and . . . (which prove) definitively for the first time that synthesis and expression of hCG, its subunits, and its fragments, is a common biochemical denomination of cancer, providing the scientific basis for studies of its prevention and/or control . . ." **(6)**

A few years earlier, a California research institute had advanced the "primordial thesis of cancer" as cutting-edge unitarianism: that cancer is nothing more or less than the capacity of an environmentally challenged natural cell to avoid cell death by "remembering" the most primordial form of life on this planet — the oxygen-less anaerobic or fermentative state — and reverting to that kind of cell. The thesis holds that the conversion is conducted through a series of repressing and de-repressing genetic events. **(7)**

Simply stated, this theory holds that *any* cell can become a cancer cell if it has been challenged with an adapt-or-die situation.

The finding of numerous "mutated" genes in the disruption of cellular machinery raises the central question:

What caused the genes to mutate, and how can the mutation be stopped or reversed?

Reducing an avalanche of information to a workable thesis:

It appears that genetic machinery may be directly or indirectly disrupted by many things (dietary excesses and deficiencies, nuclear emissions, industrial and agricultural chemicals, pollution, even mental stress and, yes, viruses) and that the damage usually involves oxidative mechanisms (*see Chapter VI*). The best defense against *all* such "organizers" of the malignant process is therefore found in the antioxidant defense system and in various aspects of immunity. The primary role players in both are nutrition and lifestyle.

This is still, again, a workable thesis only — but much more feasible than the essentially failed orthodox approach followed up to now.

Nutritional and metabolic elements in cancer management may not depend entirely on the advancing knowledge of oxidative reactions or in stimulating the body's defense against them; some may relate specifically to cancer interference by elements about whose behavior we understand little.

As a physician it has never been my primary goal to prove a theory but to save lives and reduce suffering, the essence of medicine.

I remain open, as do many of my colleagues, to further understanding the nature of cancer.

But it becomes more clear than ever that in order to understand the nature of malignancy, let alone how to control it, we must look to all aspects of mankind's civilization and that generations of living out of harmony with nature must be playing a fundamental role in the present cancer calamity.

REFERENCES

1.   Duesberg, P.H., "Human immunodeficiency virus and human immuno-deficiency syndrome: correlation but not causation." *Proc. Natl. Aca. Sci.* 86, February 1989.

2.   Morris, J.D.H., *et al.,* "Viral infection and cancer." *Lancet* 346, Sept. 16, 1995.

3.   *Ibid.*

4.   "When DNA isn't destiny." *Newsweek,* Dec. 6, 1993.

5.   *Cell,* February 1996, quoted in *US News & World Report,* March 4, 1996.

6.   Acevedo, H.F. *et al.,* "Human chorionic gonadotropin-beta subunit gene expression in cultured human fetal and cancer cells of different types and origins." *Cancer* 76:8, Oct. 15, 1995.

7.   Bradford, R.W., and Allen, H.W., *The Primordial Thesis of Cancer. Med. Hypoth.,* January 1992.

Chapter V
CANCER AND FOOD
Clues for Cause and Cure

In 1949, the American Medical Association's (AMA) Council on Pharmacy and Chemistry pompously declared, while assailing "food faddists," that

> *"[T]here is no scientific evidence whatsoever to indicate that modifications in the dietary intake of food or other nutritional essentials are of any specific value in the control of cancer."***(1)**

Forty-three years later (1992) none other than the National Cancer Institute (NCI) released the results of 156 studies — from appropriately "scientific" and "peer-reviewed" research literature — which *linked* cancer with diet.**(2)**

And two years after that (1994), the prestigious American Association for the Advancement of Science (AAAS) summarized that over the prior few decades out of 170 studies examining the roles of fruits and vegetables in cancer prevention, 129 such studies had exhibited a "significant protective effect."**(3)**

What had happened in about a half-century to so strongly vindicate both mother's insistence that we should "eat our veggies" and those dissenting natural therapy-oriented doctors who had proclaimed the diet-cancer (let alone diet-disease) linkage for many decades, often at great risk to their careers?

Simple: biochemical and epidemiological research, essentially free of the ideological and vested-interests baggage of medicine and the drug industry, had made the case for us all:

What we eat — foods, diet, nutrition — has a role to play, often a primary one, in the maintenance of wellness or the development of illness, and this is more clear in cancer than probably anywhere else, with the possible exception of the conditions bound together as "heart disease."

For me, it remains still rather incredible that, given the continual sea of new information on diet-cancer connections, the AMA itself and its oncological subdivision still remain so resistant to this concept. The vast majority of "cancer specialists" in this country (and, we might add, still the majority of standard or allopathic physicians) have little or no training in, or knowledge about, diet and disease!

This is not to place the blame entirely on the physicians, since their knowledge is dependent upon medical schools and medical journals in which nutrition is rarely, if ever, discussed.

I should know. I was trained in an orthodox medical school where, over the four years of intensive didactic teaching, exactly one week was devoted to nutrition, little, if any, of this relating diet to disease. As to medical journals, the scarcity of nutritional information is well-known.

For most metabolic/holistic physicians, proper diet is the "substrate" on which the physical aspects of a cancer prevention/cancer treatment program is based. Interestingly, this attitude, among *these* physicians, has not meaningfully changed in a century or more. It is the mainstream physicians in my opinion who are just now beginning to catch up.

While it is gratifying to watch the gradual change of concept toward the realization that what we eat has much to do with whether we actually "get" cancer, let alone how we may control or get rid of it, it is also true that our side has had more than its share of authentic faddism: there is no single one-size-fits-all anti-cancer diet, just as there is no single magic bullet to prevent, control or cure the malignant process.

But the onrush of evidence from credible epidemiological and biochemical sources is now providing a lot of clues.

Stepping back in history, until the advent of drug-oriented (allopathic) medicine toward the end of the 19th century, it was understood by virtually all healing systems that proper diet was very much involved in illness and wellness. It had a lot to do with what the medics of old called "the terrain," the natural condition of the body.

Even in the 20th century, such forward-looking researchers as Otto Warburg and Max Gerson in Germany (the latter shifting to the USA) began to place dietary connections with cancer in a Western "scientific" framework. But they, along with naturopaths and other champions of holism, remained very much on the fringe of organized medicine and were often regarded as medical heretics.

And now, their general points of view are being scientifically vindicated day by day.

Examinations of long-studied groups — national, cultural, religious — by scientific epidemiology began to turn in the overwhelming "anecdotal" evidence by the 1980s: not only cancer, but chronic disease in general, its presence, absence and/or management, has an enormous connection with what we eat.

The subject is now far too vast to be covered by one small chapter in one small book, but we can synthesize diet-cancer connections with the following observations:

THE NATURE OF WESTERN EATING HABITS HAS CHANGED

Quite aside from all other considerations, the change in eating habits in the "civilized" or Western world, where cancer and chronic disease are overwhelmingly more prominent than on the rest of the planet, has brought with it the following aspects:

(1) A reversal of the probable consumption order from primitive times. It is now relatively well recognized that primitive man ate many times more natural fruits, vegetables and grains in as raw, natural or sprouting a stage as possible, than animal fats and proteins. This was in keeping with the nature of wandering, hunter-gatherer human groups literally living off the land. Western diets, led by the appropriately acronymed Standard American Diet (SAD), have reversed the natural order: Western man consumes far more animal fats and proteins, along with stimulants, and far fewer fresh vegetables, fruits and grains. Whatever nutritious food may be produced is generally cooked to the point that all enzymes and many other nutrients are destroyed in the process (*see Chapter XII*).

(2) The removal of "seasonability" from foods. Until the 20th century, when farm mothers were both the primary-care physicians and the nutritionists/dietitians, foods were provided "in season." Anything beyond the seasonable foods was stored as a "preserve." Different foods were consumed in different seasons and other different conditions. Today, everything is literally "in season" — all the time. We can fairly well gorge ourselves at any time with foods from any season all available at the supermarket.

(3) Eating rituals are symbols of affluence. The notion, developed by the dictates of civilization, that man should eat three times a day (unlike nibbling many times per day as is the case with his nearest cousins in the food chain) has historically made the food/dining

activity a ritual of both compensation (gorging oneself during the good times to make up for the less frequent lean times) and affluence (the well-stocked larder, the well-piled dinner table indicate economic success and social achievement.)

(4) Once upon a time, it was known that the proper sequence of events, at least for most humans, was encompassed by the adage "breakfast like a king, lunch like a prince, dine like a pauper." In the Western world, we have often reversed this order — the major ritual eating activity is dinner, in which we overwhelm the body with its single largest amount of fuel during a 24-hour period and then send it into quiet repose while it figures out what to do with the excess. If it is mostly true that there should be a "major" meal of the day, biological reasoning is simple: it should be breakfast.

WE HAVE CHEMICALIZED THE FOOD SUPPLY

In the interest of a mobile, technological, ever-changing population of the affluent, not only have supermarkets replaced the "seasonability" of foods, but the food-processing industry — the number-one profit-taker on Wall Street **(4)** — has, in the name of convenience, marketability, preservation, conservation, seduction and, yes, greed, altered the food supply by chemicalizing it.

Estimates on what has been done to our foods — to "keep" them, color them, buffer them, enhance their appearance, taste, commercial appeal, etc. — are that, beginning at about the second decade of this century, between 10,000 and 50,000 synthetic chemicals of all kinds have been inserted directly into the food supply or into the animals and soils which will produce that supply. These range from artificial hormones to fatten farm animals and poultry and to enhance bulk and egg-laying to compounds used to color, preserve and make more visually pleasing any number of foodstuffs.

The concept of "enriched" foods thus developed earlier in this century. In bread, the very feeble staff of life these days, many natural nutrients have been removed or destroyed by food processing. When a few of them are replaced, the product is said to be "enriched," as awesome an oxymoron as can be industrially conceived.

Food processing, not a sinister plot but an industrial response to the needs of a mobile, affluent society, by altering the intrinsic nature of foods in removing many natural nutrients and adding new ones, has thus provided the human body with many chemical compounds not natural to its biological experience. If one adds to these the synthetic compounds available as antibiotics, steroids and other medications it is safe to assume that humans, particularly Westerners, are now exposed to upwards of 100,000 synthetic compounds for which human experience has no ancestral memory. This does not mean that they are all bad — only that the body doesn't know what to do with them. It should not surprise anyone that immunological disorders unknown a few decades ago, and runaway cancer rates, are now so prominent in our "Western civilization."

DEPLETED SOILS AND DEPLETED FOODS
MEAN DEPLETED PEOPLE

The industrial revolution in agriculture in North America — the replacement of small family farms with huge corporate ones answering the insatiable demands for "more food" of an ever-hungrier, ever-growing population — has added tens of thousands of chemicals to the soil and subsoil in the name of crop enhancement as well as crop protection (pesticides, herbicides, insecticides). This has resulted in such notorious problems as the "heart disease belt" in the South, whose major features are depletion of trace-mineral selenium from the soil and the consumption of trace mineral-depleted foods grown in such soil.

The switch from "natural" to industrial farming, warned about years ago, has hence brought chemical mayhem upon us as a major ingredient in chronic disease and cancer.

DIETARY AND NUTRIENT RECOMMENDATIONS
ARE A FARCE

Economic considerations are behind the US industrial/governmental establishment's intermittent pronouncements about "recommended daily allowances" of nutrients (vitamins, minerals, enzymes, essential fatty acids) and "balanced dietary guidelines" which are constantly revised.

That the establishment cheats overwhelmingly on this issue was made particularly clear in 1993 when it surfaced that a federal government report in 1971 which had found that a majority of the nation's health ills were connected with diet and that their solutions could be found in good nutrition had been suppressed for an amazing 22 years! **(5)**

Other volumes (I heartily recommend co-author Culbert's and the late Dr. Harold Harper's) have gone into great detail about how the "recommended daily allowances" and "dietary guidelines" were established as adjuncts to the food-processing industry and bear no resemblance to biological reason. **(6,7,8)**

Of the existing "dietary guidelines" for the "four food groups," there might be some value in them if the foods were from natural sources. As it is, simply balancing the levels of vegetables, fruits, grains and meats is only meaningful if we know the *source* of them.

In just one key food area — carbohydrates — we may be faced with the gravest calamity of all. "Unnatural" or "oxidized" refined carbohydrates, the "junk foods" of several generations, may in fact be setting the stage for the blood sugar disturbances (glucose metabolism dysfunction) which, together with the problem of depleted antioxidants in general (*see Chapter VII*), constitute the bedrock on which chronic disease in general, and cancer in particular, is built.

In my practice, and that of many others, a substantial percentage of my cancer patients have pre-existing or concurrent diabetic or pre-diabetic conditions. The overlaps between refined carbohydrates, obesity, aging, cancer and death are now far too numerous to be ignored.

'THE POOR PEOPLE'S DIET'

Whether described as "mostly alkaline" or "the dietary of protein deprivation," wherever the diets of poor people around the world are studied, they absolutely correlate with the statistically low incidence, or actual absence, of chronic disease, headed by cancer.

Over-simplifying the issue (since dietary variations also relate to cultural, racial, and probably genetic patterns), the poor people's diet, so bereft of chronic disease, is made up largely of the following components:

More vegetables and fruits in as fresh, raw or sprouting a condition as possible; more natural, unrefined, wild grains; *no* stimulants (as in colas, teas and coffee); *no* refined carbohydrates — yet there may be many "reduced" or natural ones; and far less animal fat and animal protein.

That is, a return to the primitive eating habits of early man.

In this book we look at some specific elements (vitamins, minerals, enzymes, phytochemicals) that may relate to cancer either directly or indirectly. But single-nutrient theories aside, the above-described diet is in alignment with the reality that abundant natural nutrients have direct and indirect anti-cancer effects, immune system-modulating properties (*see Chapter VI*) and aid in detoxification.

This is usually why metabolic therapists, even though they may prefer or promote one particular item (laetrile, say, or vitamin C, or Carnivora, or co-enzyme Q10, or any number of herbal combinations), almost always accompany such a therapy with an eating program very similar to the poor people's diet.

We see in this a synergism between many useful, natural ingredients — not "magic bullets" to "destroy tumors."

Aspects of the very same diet which helps prevent chronic disease hence can be marshaled to treat, control or cure such diseases — a restatement of the old medical adage "that which prevents, also cures."

REFERENCES

1. Quoted in Culbert, M.L., *Medical Armageddon.* San Diego CA: C & C Communications, 1995.
2. *The Choice,* XIX:1, 1994.
3. Culbert, M.L., *op. cit.*
4. McGee, C.T., *Heart Frauds.* Coeur d'Alene ID: MediPress, 1993.
5. *Human Nutrition Report No. 2: Benefits from Human Nutrition Research.* Washington DC: US Dept. of Agriculture, 1971.
6. Culbert, *op. cit.*
7. Harper, H.W., and Culbert, M.L., *How You Can Beat the Killer Diseases.* New Rochelle NY: Arlington House, 1977.
8. Culbert, M.L., *What the Medical Establishment Won't Tell You that Could Save Your Life.* Norfolk VA: Donning, 1983.

Chapter VI
IMMUNE MODULATION
Building Host Defense

It is largely thanks to the AIDS pandemic beginning in the 1980s that we now know a lot more about the interlock of actions, cells and organs usually referred to simply as "the immune system" — a somewhat misleading term inasmuch as all portions of the body's ability to protect itself against disease more properly fit into the broader term "host defense."

Since a good deal of the malignant process is indeed strongly related to a depressed or "ineffective" host defense system, and because much of the failure of standard or orthodox therapies (chemotherapy, radiation, surgery) against cancer is due to their suppressive effect on this system, the importance of immunity has risen to prominence in Western medicine.

While it is not correct to say that *all* cancer is always related to immune depression (for some cancer seems to be associated with immune excitation— an "overactive" system) it is generally correct to say that the malignant condition prospers in a state of profound immune *dysregulation*, a point strongly made by one of the authors (Culbert) in CFS (chronic fatigue syndrome) and URS (universal reactor syndrome). **(1,2)**

It is now understood that many of the natural modalities long employed against cancer are useful against the malignant process because of their ability to help regulate a de-regulated or dysfunctional host defense system. Numerous nutrients and other natural factors may play roles, often decisive, in correcting defects in what we call "the immune system":

Rather than continuing to refer vaguely to the "immune system," it should be helpful to be more specific as to what elements make up that system, a few of which are:

- *Lymphocytes*: These are types of white blood cells directly involved in the primary immune response. By this is meant the body's initial reaction to disease, or the first line of defense. There are several specialized types of lymphocytes, including the T-lymphocytes, so named for their dependency on, and activation by, the thymus gland.

Several types of T-cells interact with one another and with other elements of the immune system, assuring a coordinated attack upon cancer cells.

There are "memory" T-cells which have the capacity to recognize abnormal cells such as cancer cells, pre-cancer or degenerating cells, and these in turn alert the "troops," mainly other T-cells, particularly the "helper" (T4) T-cells which in turn activate more of the "troops" by giving instructions to attack the enemy.

The primary attack force consists of the NK or "natural killer" cells which, taking their orders from helper T-cells and others, directly attack and destroy cancer cells, even at very early stages.

So-called "suppressor" (T8) T-cells slow down the process after the enemy has been destroyed to prevent the destructive process from going too far, and possibly damaging normal tissue.

- *Macrophages*: Another member of the first line of defense team, the macrophage is derived from another type of white blood cell, the granulocyte. Literally "big eaters," these cells are our "scavengers," and, like memory T-cells, have the capacity to recognize and seek out abnormal cells, bacteria, viruses, or anything that "appears" to them to be aberrant or out of place — of course including cancer cells. The macrophages are then able to surround, attack and ingest that abnormal something and carry it away.

- *Cytokines*: These hormone-like "messengers" are polypeptide protein complexes that are the means of communication between the various organs involved in the immune response, such as the brain and central nervous system, thymus, and spleen, allowing them to "talk" to the blood-cell elements under discussion here.

- *Lymphokines*: Chemical messengers like the cytokines, these more specifically facilitate communication between the different types of lymphocytes, helping to provide for a highly coordinated immune response. The interleukins and interferons fit into this category.

- *B-Lymphocytes*: So named because of their origin from bones or *bursae*, this subset or subdivision of the lymphocyte family has the ability to produce specific antibodies against specific diseases. Every disease-causing virus and bacteria is recognized by the body as being a foreign antigen, calling for the production of protein substances called antibodies which are specific to one disease antigen only.

- *Immunoglobulins:* These protein substances are produced by B-lymphocytes and their descendants, the plasma cells. They consist of a huge array of protein complexes which are immunologically active. The B-cells are able to "recognize" disease organisms — viruses, bacteria, allergens, and other foreign substances — and then produce specific antibodies able to oppose such invaders. The diversity of this system is enormous, since it is able to recognize and react to an almost infinite number of antigens, foreign substances, and different types of disease organisms.

In addition to infectious disease organisms, degenerating cells originating within the body are also regarded by the B-cells as antigens or something to be destroyed.

Consequently, when previously normal cells break down or degenerate into pre-cancer cells or early cancer cells, the sentinels of the body produce antibodies which are highly specific to these cells and attach to them, thus forming an "immune complex," and then facilitate their destruction.

This portion of the immune system is referred to as the "second line of defense," but it is coordinated with the first line of defense since it calls upon the macrophages to destroy the immune complexes which include the abnormal cells.

- *Complement System*: This third line of defense consists of a vast array of proteins which provide another powerful weapon of defense against disease, and a backup to the antibody system. After the alarm is sounded by the "sentinels" of the immune system, and after antibodies attach themselves to the diseased cells, signals (by means of peptides/cytokines) contact the complement "soldiers" which then attach themselves to the antibodies ("the good guys") and the whole complex is destroyed.

- *Reticuloendothelial System*: The bedrock of all aspects of immunity, this system includes spleen, liver, and bone marrow, and its functions include the production of all white blood cells and synthesis of many proteins involved in the "immune system."

The purpose of having so many systems within the "immune system," of course, is ultimately the safety of the host. In the event of failure or inadequacy of one "swat team," there are several more to come to the rescue.

To the extent that any part of any one of these systems is defective, any substance which helps overcome the defect may be referred to as an "immune enhancer." To the extent that certain substances may depress parts of immunity (e.g., excess T8 cells) the same may be called "immune suppressors."

To the extent that some substances, and certainly most toxic drugs, may damage or lower immune response, the same may also be called "immune suppressors."

In cancer, as in chronic disease in general, and given the growing reality that it is immune *dysregulation* — rather than simply immune depression or immune excitation — many natural substances are now better classed as "non-specific immune modulators" because their total effects seem to "balance" a damaged host-defense apparatus even though the specific ways in which they do this are not fully understood.

Strangely, as of this late date (mid-1990s) Western medical orthodoxy still insists there is no known way to boost a flagging "immune system" other than the administration of toxic (and expensive) synthetic proteins, particularly of interferons and interleukins, the record for which is spotty at best.

It is interesting to note that the conventional dosages for both alpha-interferon and interleukin-2 are in the neighborhood of 90 million units per day, a level which is often accompanied by serious side effects, including death. However, some of us practicing holistic or alternative medicine have found that much lower doses, such as three million units, carry no side effects, cost much less, and have a favorable "tonifying" effect on the immune system, adding to the overall immune activation provided by other supplements, modalities, and immune-enhancing substances.

So it seems that cancer orthodoxy remains committed to the "overkill" school of thought — i.e., if a little is good, more is better. Mainstream medicine, while more or less on the right track with the interleukins and interferons, since they are basically natural immune boosters, continues to have a large blind spot, for the most part, in the area of immune enhancement.

Yet metabolic and holistic doctors for generations have seen in many nutrients the capability of helping restore or balance an impaired host defense.

Many of the standard nutrients now used against chronic disease, captained by vitamins A, C, E, and the B complex, have, among many aspects, the capability of serving as non-specific immune modulators.

For example, a deficiency of vitamin B6 or pyridoxine may contribute to defective T-lymphocyte formation which in turn leads to inadequate immune responses to a host of maladies, including cancer. Vitamin B6 is, along with other nutrients, including certain essential fatty acids, essential to the production of the hormone-like prostaglandin E1, which in turn is necessary for normal thymus function and regulation of T-cells. A deficiency of folic acid, another B vitamin, is also correlated to depressed host defense.

Not until recently have the links between essential fatty acids (EFA) and immunity become better understood with the calamity of AIDS as the open door.

For it can now be said that deficiencies of certain EFAs, as well as the alteration of some of them by the hydrogenation technique of modern food processing (with the consequent introduction of abnormal *trans* fatty acids into humans), play some intriguing roles in immune dysregulation. **(3,4,5)**

Recent research has thus tended to bolster the assertion by M.I. Gurr in 1983 that lipid (blood fat)-immune response studies

". . . illustrate once more the principle that PG [prostaglandins] and EFA [essential fatty acids] may modify immune function according to a bell-shaped dose-response relationship and should now be regarded as modulators of immune function rather than as simple inhibitors." **(6)**

Such observations help explain why some metabolic therapists have added such EFA-containing substances as evening primrose oil and fish oils to overall programs. Cis-linoleic acid, arachadonic acid, gamma-linolenic acid and eicosapentanoic acid are the nutritive elements of major importance here.

Among the minerals, which (as is the case for zinc and selenium) are also useful as antioxidants (*see Chapter VII*) against the cancer process, the all-purpose germanium has both antioxidant *and* immune cell-activation properties and also enhances the production of natural interferon in the body.

Since the thymus gland, which gradually atrophies as we get older, is usually thought of as the immune-system "master switch," a key processor of immune cells, keeping it boosted or bolstered has long been seen as an essential part of a total therapy.

Zinc deficiency and, probably, EFA deficiency, are implicated in thymus atrophy in both animal models and in malnourished human children. Since both AIDS and cancer frequently share the trait of malnutrition, the role of both deficiencies in immune enhancement becomes clearer. **(7,8)**

The thymus produces some 60 different hormone-like proteins called *peptides* or *polypeptides* (descriptions of arrangements of amino acids, the building blocks of protein) which act as chemical messengers throughout the body. In cancer, for example, the messengers instruct the T-cells in general and "killer T-cells" in particular to seek out and destroy viruses, other disease-causing organisms, and, at some stage, cancer cells.

Hence, both extracts of the thymus gland, and even oral preparations of ground-up thymus glands, have been and are frequently used in a total anti-cancer program.

There are also various thymus polypeptides and peptides which, on their own, have been found useful against malignancy.

Among these are the controversial "antineoplastons" developed decades ago by the embattled Polish emigre physician/biochemist Stanislaw Burzynski in Houston, Texas (*see Chapter XIII*).

After years of meticulous study and research this gifted scientist was able to isolate, from human urine, several peptides proven to be effective in controlling the growth of certain "forms" of cancer. Considering them to be part of a "parallel immune system," he started using what he called antineoplastons as non-toxic cancer therapy. This stimulated virtually as big a controversy as laetrile had at an earlier time (*see Chapter IX*).

Some peptides are produced by the spleen and brain as well as by the thymus gland and some are made by the white blood cells themselves. The better known interferons and interleukins are peptides, and they can be stimulated *naturally* within the body.

These "messenger chemicals," referred to earlier in connection with the brain, thymus and other organs as "talking" to T-cells and others, are all peptides or polypeptides essential to the integrated organization of body components we call the immune system. Included are the lymphokines and cytokines by which lymphocytes and other cells "talk" to each other and receive instructions from, say, the thymus, whenever the threat of disease calls for the alerting and organizing of the host defense.

Some peptides act as neurotransmitters, carrying messages from the hypothalamus at the base of the brain to the thymus and other organs, triggering the release of other chemicals — usually peptides — which then bring on the whole cascade of reactions we refer to as the immune response.

Dr. Burzynski and others believe that some of these important substances are lacking in the cancer patient, which would account for the fact that so many such patients respond so well to these natural body chemicals. While I have no experience with the particular peptides isolated and synthesized by Dr. Burzynski, I have found similar substances to be very useful additions to our arsenal of immune-enhancing, cancer-fighting weapons.

There are other aspects of host defense which at first blush seem to have little to do with immunology.

A good night's sleep, for example, may be as important in an overall therapy as the proper use of a polypeptide or a vitamin or a mineral. Adequate rest and relaxation provide total-body metabolic benefits to the patient even in the absence of a total understanding of just how they "work."

A disturbance in sleep patterns has provided part of the reason for using one of the more recent breakthrough items in natural therapy — melatonin, a hormone produced by the mysterious pineal gland in the center of the brain that the Ancients thought of as the seat of the soul. We know that the response of the body to light is largely a function of the pineal gland, and that sleep disturbances may have a good deal to do with confusing signals from light — as when an intercontinental jet traveler passes through many time zones in one trip, thus "fooling" the body (and the pineal) by altering its response to natural light.

It is now known that excesses or deficiencies in hormones produced by the adrenal glands have multiple effects on the body, and that such disturbances are common in, for example, AIDS and CFS while not infrequent in cancer. For this reason, endocrinological (hormone) balancing is a frequent part of a total program for chronic disease, whether accomplished by individual hormone applications (as in the case of DHEAS or DHEA for the adrenals) or even by live-cell or cellular therapy (*see Chapter XIII*).

Hormones, the master chemical messengers of the body, impact on many aspects of biological activity, including all portions of what is generally called "the immune system" and hence are interwoven with that system.

For some, the route to good health, and the basis of a sound treatment program above all other specifics, is encompassed by the three essentials of building and protecting host defense:

DETOXIFICATION, through proper diet, fasting, juicing, restoration of normal bacterial flora to the intestine with "probiotics" such as acidophilus, enemas, colonics, and intravenous approaches, such as chelation therapy, and/or other techniques.

RESTORATION of normal physiologic functions and replacement of nutritional and hormonal deficiencies contributing to whatever abnormal or inadequate body functions exist. This includes restoration of peace of mind, as well as that of the physical body.

MODULATION of immune function, usually enhancement of such function in the case of cancer, using many of the foregoing substances and modalities to accomplish this.

Whatever other specifics in a program (necessary surgery, for example, and/or administration of disease-fighting chemicals), the foregoing "Big 3" in building host defense must be the foundation.

REFERENCES

1.   Culbert, M.L., *CFS: Conquering the Crippler.* San Diego CA: C & C Communications, 1993.

2.   Culbert, M.L., *Toward a Unified Theory of Immune Dysfunction and its Management.* Chula Vista CA: Bradford Research Institute, 1992.

3.   Horrobin, D. F., *et al.,* "The nutritional regulation of T lymphocyte function." *Med. Hypoth. V,* 1979.

4.   Holman, R.T., and Aes-Jorgenson, E., "Effects of trans fatty isomers upon essential fatty acid deficiency in rats." *Proc. Soc. Exp. Biol. Med.* 93, 1956.

5.   Booyens, J., and van der Merwe, C.F., "Chronic arachidonic acid eicosanoid imbalance: a common feature in coronary artery disease, hypercholesterolemia, cancer and other important diseases." *Med. Hypoth.* 18, 1965.

6.   Gurr, M.I., "The role of lipids in the regulation of the immune system." *Prog. Lipid. Res.* 22, 1983.

7.   Horrobin, *op. cit.*

8.   Golden, M.H.N., *et al.,* "Zinc and immunocompetence in protein-energy malnutrition." *Lancet* 2, 1978.

Chapter VII
ANTIOXIDANTS AGAINST CANCER:
The Oxidology Revolution

Perhaps it is simple irony that a central fact regarding health and disease in animals on earth is that while they cannot live for more than a few minutes without oxygen, the way in which their organisms "handle" the life-sustaining gas probably has more to do than any other single item with the maintenance of health or the onset of disease.

Oxidation is the primary mechanism by which the body turns food into energy and supplies power to all of our muscles, organs and other tissues.

Yet it has a dark side — even though it is one of the most basic and necessary of human biochemical processes, not all oxidation is desirable and some of it can become damaging and disease-producing, particularly in the realm of chronic disease and cancer.

In terms of oxidation, there is, at the cellular (and even submicroscopic) level, a continuing battlefield of life and death.

In the last two decades of this century the explosion of knowledge regarding the role of oxygen (itself and its breakdown products) in health and disease has been so great that at least one California group decided that the subspecialty needed its own name — *oxidology*— which is already being adopted into foreign languages. **(1)**

Oxidology research from various angles has implicated oxygen byproduct damage to cellular DNA, protein and blood fats (lipids) as a major contributor to chronic disease, degenerative conditions, immune system dysregulation, brain dysfunction, cataracts, other conditions, and aging itself. **(2,3,4,5)**

Whether grouped under "free radical pathology," "oxidative techniques" or "management of reactive oxygen species" we are dealing with oxidology. At this writing, the components of a vast array of chronic and systemic conditions ranging from heart and circulatory diseases to immune disorders, and increasingly in all aspects of cancer, make it ever more clear that virtually *all* chronic and metabolic disturbances, and to some extent even all pathology in general, are inextricably linked to the way the body utilizes oxygen.

Much has been written in recent years about free radical pathology as our knowledge of this phenomenon continues to grow.

Every stable molecule consists of a proton (positively charged particle) in its center, with paired electrons (negatively charged) circling in orbit around the central particle. Whenever, in the course of the thousands of oxidation reactions occurring daily in the body, a molecule loses one of its electrons, it becomes a "free radical," unstable and a "seeker of electrons."

Nature always inclines toward stability, so these unstable molecules attempt to react with electrons of other molecules, representing a threat to every tissue in the body.

The increased understanding of free radical pathology and how it contributes to the causation of disease has provided unexpected validation of something previously regarded as wholly unorthodox — namely, the use of nutrition and diet against cancer.

This is because so many nutritive elements (vitamins, minerals, amino acids, hormone-like substances, various phytochemicals) are, among other things, *antioxidants*; that is, they "scavenge" or "inhibit" the activity of excess toxic oxygen byproducts, for which "free radicals" is the better-known term even though it is more precise to call them reactive oxygen toxic species (ROTS), an acronym descriptive of their action.

For example, if for no other reason than their capacity to scavenge ROTS, there is now a solidly, biochemically established reason to utilize beta-carotene, vitamins C and E, laetrile, selenium and zinc as therapies against chronic disease, very much including cancer. Concerning the latter, it is now recognized that the malignant process, including its metastatic (spread-capable) function, is deeply involved in the prodigious production of reactive oxygen molecules (ROTS). **(6)**

Free radicals or ROTS may be produced by such external factors as cigarette smoke, industrial chemicals and radiation. Internally, they may be produced as byproducts of aerobic cellular respiration, the inflammatory process (in which they often serve a highly useful purpose) and even the activity of immune system cells. Some five percent of the oxygen we breathe is converted to ROTS, or free radicals. And the body's very own "master free radical producer" itself is none other than natural hydrogen peroxide (H_2O_2), elicited by the host defense mechanism in small quantities for very specific purposes.

The "oxygen free radicals" are those most implicated in health and disease.

As the body processes or utilizes the oxygen without which it cannot live, it is producing harmful byproducts which can help provoke its death — so the internal fail-safe mechanism of superoxide dismutase, glutathione peroxidase and catalase enzymes comes into play. These, in turn, are largely dependent on trace minerals, particularly zinc, copper and selenium.

Other nutrients we refer to as antioxidants must be present to help "handle" the unstable free radicals. These include vitamin C, which the human species can only secure from exogenous (outside the body) sources, beta-carotene (the vitamin A "precursor") and vitamin E (the tocopherols). Adequate levels of glutathione, proteins and uric acid, and sufficient balance of the immune system (whose macrophage and neutrophil cells deliver their lethal attack on foreign invaders by generating ROTS), must also be maintained.

These highly reactive ROTS molecules, or, more precisely, portions of molecules, are known to attack unprotected cells in several areas. Probably the most important target in the cell is the DNA — the template determining the exact nature of the next generation of cells — which, when damaged, leads to the development of abnormal cells leading in turn to cancer or other degenerative disease.

One key researcher, Bruce Ames, has estimated that cellular DNA is oxidatively "hit" at least 10,000 times a day in every human — even every presumably healthy human. **(7)**

Another component of the cell susceptible to free radical attack is the lysosome, a small sac within the cell containing a powerful enzyme called lysozyme. When the sac or membrane of this tiny compartment is penetrated by free radicals or ROTS particles, the enzyme is "spilled" into the cell, resulting in self-digestion and extensive destruction of the cell. The consequence of this process is either a dead cell or an abnormal cell, which often evolves into a cancer cell.

The cellular enzymes are there to patch up the damage, depending, of course, on the total nutritional environment of the body, particularly as it ages, quite aside from its own inherited stability.

There is increasing evidence that virtually *all* cellular damage is "mediated" through oxidative/antioxidant tension, whether that damage be initiated by harmful industrial chemical overload, exposure to radiation, or some other exogenous factor. Theoretically, mother nature's failsafe mechanism for survival of the human race is the ability of the body to manage constant free-radical attack internally (through the antioxidant enzyme system) up to early middle age.

There is some indication that as aging advances internal antioxidant enzyme defense tapers off. That is to say, the "first line of defense" against chronic disease may be diminished by advancing age itself. If the "second team" — the nutritional factors which support the precarious balance between oxidation/antioxidant activity — is not present or is inadequately present then chronic disease and premature aging result.

Increasing research suggests that the same chain of events leads to the development of cancer (*see Chapter IV*), a situation in which ROTS damage, among other factors, has initiated a chain of genetic events which will cause a natural cell to revert to a fermentative, anaerobic (primordial) condition. **(8,9,10)**

Happily, the same advances in oxidology suggest avenues of defense and attack:

It is often the antioxidant (that is, free radical-scavenging) capability of specific nutrients which provides an anti-cancer attack at the cellular and subcellular level.

If one has sufficient vitamins, minerals, amino acids, flavonoids and numerous other nutrients one's own antioxidant defense system is enhanced. This suggests defense not only against the malignant process but against degenerative disease in general, irrespective of the immune system-modulating effects of some of the same nutrients.

In the simplest terms, a wide range of nutrients found primarily in fresh fruits and vegetables provides heavy armor against internal oxidative damage by free radicals and ROTS and thus a protection against overt cancer irrespective of any genetic predisposition to that process.

The modern breakthrough in oxidology now provides a sound biochemical rationale for a large portion of what some have called the "alkaline" eating program or the "diet of privation" of the poor people of the world, who, by depending on freshly grown fruits, vegetables and grains and far less animal fat and protein, and by living a lifestyle far freer of ROTS-causing chemicals, are continually enhancing their internal antioxidant defense mechanism.

The health of every cell in the body is the key to the health of the body itself. Each one of our trillions of cells must breathe, excrete, take in oxygen and glucose and divide normally. If the computer of each cell, cellular DNA, is protected against internal free-radical attack, the likelihood of preventing cancer, let alone chronic disease in general, is greatly enhanced.

Metabolic doctors no longer have to keep their heads down as they prescribe — as I do — vitamins C and E, beta-carotene, glutathione, the amino acids cysteine and methionine, the trace minerals zinc and selenium, germanium, and the recently described proanthocyanidins (Pycnogenol), the pineal hormone melatonin, or a host of nutrients and herbs all of which are "anticancer agents" in that, whatever else they may be doing, they are "scavenging" the toxic oxygen byproducts called ROTS or free radicals.

There is an interesting other side to the oxidative/antioxidant equation:

Oxidative agents are those factors which generate atomic oxygen and whose primary internal manifestation is hydrogen peroxide. This, as well as ozone (O_3), a gas, and industrial compounds of chlorine oxides, such as Dioxychlor, have been found useful at various levels of anti-cancer therapeutics by exploiting cancer's well-known aversion to oxygen. All such oxidative agents are also used in the "alternative" armamentarium as anti-infective and antiviral agents because of their manifest ability to attack cell wall-deficient structures.

Both hydrogen peroxide (H_2O_2) and ozone (O_3) have been promoted as magic-bullet "cures" of cancer which, of course, they are not, but I am aware that intratumoral infusions of ozone into accessible tumors may indeed bring about local destruction of cancer masses. This does not equate with the "curing" of cancer but does suggest an essentially non-surgical, non-toxic approach to dealing with an accessible malignant growth.

But caution must be sounded concerning the overuse of H_2O_2 and O_3. Both may ultimately lead, through the "free radical cascade," to the generation of free radicals. Unless adequate antioxidant protection accompanies the use of oxidative agents, the over-utilization of such agents, whose end result is the production of ROTS, may be a case of robbing Peter to pay Paul.

Orthodox oncology is beginning to grasp the importance of the antioxidant nutrients as — at the very least — "adjuvant therapy" in cancer.

Since the common cancer treatments of chemotherapy and radiation actually are "oxidative" in action, it was long held that the administration of antioxidants would reduce their effectiveness. Yet clinical studies have indicated that high-dose administration of antioxidants enhances such standard therapies (11,12) and these have been consistent with my own clinical observations. This is another reason why some orthodox practitioners are at least beginning to look at the broad area of nutrients against the malignant process.

As we have seen (*see Chapter IV*), cancer cells are formed on a daily basis in every one of us, by the thousands, but this does not mean that we will all develop cancer, thanks to our awesome defense system and all of its many backup protective features.

A thorough understanding of free radical pathology and its interaction with the immune system is of major importance in designing any health care program, whether it be one of prevention or disease management.

REFERENCES

1. Bradford, R.W., *et al., Oxidology: the Study of Reactive Oxygen Toxic Species (ROTS) and Their Metabolism in Health and Disease.* Los Altos CA: the Bradford Foundation, 1985.

2. Ames, B.N., *et al.,* "Oxidants, antioxidants and the degenerative diseases of aging." *Proc. Natl. Acad. Sci. USA* 90, 1993.

3. Jenner, P., "Oxidative damage in neurodegenerative disease." *Lancet,* Sept. 17, 1994.

4. Grisham, N.B., "Oxidants and free radicals in inflammatory bowel disease." *Lancet,* Sept. 24, 1994.

5. Reiter, R.J., *et al.,* "A review of the evidence supporting melatonin's role as an antioxidant." *J. Pineal Res.* 18, 1995.

6. Bradford, *op. cit.*

7. Ames, *op. cit.*

8. Cerutti, B.A. "Oxy-radicals and cancer." *Lancet,* Sept. 24, 1994.

9. Bradford, R.W. and Allen, H.W., *The Primordial Thesis of Cancer. Med. Hypoth.* January 1992.

10. Hietanen, E., *et al.,* "Diet and oxidative stress in breast, colon, and prostate cancer patients: a case-control study." *Eur. J. Clin. Nutr.* 48, 1994.

11. Quillin, Patrick, "Adjuvant nutrition in cancer treatment." *J. Adv. in Med. 8:3,* 1995.

12. Jaakkola, K., *et al.,* "Treatment with antioxidant and other nutrients in combination with chemotherapy and irradiation in patients with small cell lung cancer." *Antican. Res.* 12, 1992.

Chapter VIII
NUTRIENTS AGAINST CANCER
Weapons from Mother Nature's Vast Pharmacopeia

Over the past quarter century there has been a virtual explosion of knowledge regarding the use of foods and nutritive elements against chronic disease in general and cancer in particular.

During this time, many physicians and researchers in the field have maintained that food and diet are mainstays in health and wellness and that it would behoove the Western scientific establishment to pay more organized attention to certain *elements* within foods which play specific roles in the fight against cancer.

There have been many valid investigations of the better-known vitamins, minerals and enzymes which have confirmed their direct and indirect anti-cancer properties.

After literally being in the closet of conventional cancer medicine for most of this century, vitamins A, C, E, minerals such as zinc, germanium and selenium, factors such as co-enzyme Q10, chlorophyll, quercitin, the flavonoids, digestive enzymes, parts of the B-vitamin family, have emerged as — among their many other qualities — preventers of the malignant process. To many of us — and this is far from unanimous, even among holistic physicians — that which helps to prevent cancer should also be useful in fighting the disease.

In the vitamin category, most Americans are now aware of Linus Pauling's work with vitamin C against the common cold, but fewer are aware of Pauling's and Ewan Cameron's research, and that of Irwin Stone, which demonstrated the effectiveness of vitamin C (as ascorbic acid or ascorbate) against cancer.[1,2]

They showed that this major vitamin, which the human must acquire from outside sources, has an inhibitory effect on the invasiveness of cancer cells while having several positive effects on the immune response.

The ascorbates appear to have the ability to selectively kill tumor cells in a manner similar to the chemotherapeutic drugs used by conventional oncologists.(3) Unlike chemotherapy, however, vitamin C actually *enhances* those parts of the immune system that are highly active against cancer, notably the natural killer (NK) cells.(4)

In clinical practice, ascorbic acid or ascorbates given in high doses, usually intravenously, have an almost immediate positive effect on the cancer patient's feeling of well-being. Yet medical orthodoxy raised almost as much objection and opposition to the use of this nutrient against cancer as it had to the use of amygdalin (laetrile or vitamin B17), also a vitamin-like substance (*see Chapter IX*).

Vitamin A and its precursor, beta-carotene , have been subjected to more cancer research than any other nutrient. While the results have been mixed, there is far more favorable than unfavorable evidence in this area. Vitamin A is essential to a healthy immune system and provides extra resistance to cancer by stimulating and enhancing the activity of natural killer T-cells against cancer cells. (5,6,7) Scattered research indicates that vitamin A provides protection against certain specific "types" of cancer, particularly those involving lung, skin and other epithelial surfaces.

In a study of men with a conventionally untreatable "form" of lung cancer, treated with vitamin A or cis-retinoic acid (a form of vitamin A), all showed substantial improvement after 15 months.(8)

In an Italian study it was found that the use of a combination of vitamins A, C and E resulted in fewer malignant cells arising in people at high risk for colorectal cancer following rectal surgery for adenoma (benign tumors). Patients in this study received relatively high doses of vitamin A — 25,000 to 50,000 units per day for months — and yet they showed no evidence of liver damage or other complications.(9)

Squamous metaplasia, or conversion of normal surface cells to cancer cells, can be reversed by vitamin A or its derivatives for a number of conditions. Some research indicates that vitamin A inhibits the *promotion* of cancer, while beta-carotene (vitamin A's precursor) inhibits the *initiation* of cancer.

This suggests that vitamin A may actually play a more active role in cancer treatment than beta-carotene.(10) These findings are consistent with my clinical observations with the use of this all-important vitamin.

Supplementation with vitamin E has been associated with reduced risk of certain cancers**(11,12)** and pre-cancerous conditions.**(13)**

Vitamin E and its relatives, the tocopherols, have been shown to have a positive effect on immune response and resistance to disease, both in animals**(14)** and humans.**(15,16)**

A deficiency of vitamin E results, among other things, in impairment of T-cell function**(17)** and decreased scavenging activity by the macrophages (big eaters),**(15)** both functions being necessary to the body's ability to effectively fight cancer (*see Chapter VI*). Both of these immune functions are reversible with vitamin E supplementation.**(18,19,20)**

The renewed attention to vitamins, minerals and other food factors has been accompanied by a widespread revival of interest in herbs. After all, herbalism, aside from religious ritual and the laying on of hands, is the oldest form of medicine in the world and the foundation of most medicines of today. With this revival has come intensive inquiry into herbs and their ingredients, and attempts to discover how they "work" in preventing or treating certain cancers.

The immense cultural heritage of Native Americans and Mesoamericans is now looked upon in a new light. A great deal of information has been uncovered, albeit it largely anecdotal, on the widespread effects of herbs against cancer and other diseases, particularly among the North American Indians.**(21,22)**

A political event also helped spur the renewed interest in herbs: the USA's "opening to China," the medical aspect of which first brought the millennia-old practices of acupuncture and acupressure to Western "scientific" attention. Right behind this, China's 4,000-year experience with herbs could hardly be ignored.

Within a few years, the American orthodox cancer establishment had officially "cleared" two Chinese herbs and/or their extracts (*astragalus* and *lingustrum*) as anti-cancer fighters in the American medical marketplace. But this has been only the tip of a gigantic iceberg of information flowing Eastward from mainland China.

In an excellent 1995 assessment which attempted to place natural anti-cancer modalities, including herbs, within the parameters of Western "science," John Boik reviewed a startling 375 individual Chinese herbs and some 44 combinations of these, many of which were found to have direct or indirect uses in a total management program of cancer. This is the most extensive overview of useful Chinese herbs of which we are aware.(23)

Earlier, investigators Eric J. Lien and W.Y. Li surveyed some 120 species of Chinese plants and herbs, most of which had various uses against cancer.(24)

"Uses" here refers to a very broad base of activities, many of which are found in the same herbs. As poultices, gels, powders, liquids, pills, or consumed naturally (leaves, stems, roots, or tops) or injectable preparations, "uses" may include everything from such activity as "biological response modification" to the wide world of "non-specific immune modulation," to immune stimulation, immune depression, hormone-pool modification, bile secretion stimulation, blood cleansing, antiseptic, anti-inflammatory and other actions aside from direct interference with cancer cell replication.

Knowledge of the better-known European and North American herbs has led to such breakthroughs as the semisynthetic drug Ukrain (*see Chapter XI*), derived from the honorable old greater celandine herb, to such modern-day combinations as the Hoxsey herbal tonics, which now have sufficient pedigree to be established as useful in numerous cancer cases,(25) and even Essiac tea, the historic contribution by the late Rene Caisse, a Canadian nurse, to cancer "cures" from North American Indian sources.(26)

Research has isolated such useful anti-cancer modalities as Iscador from the mistletoe herb (*Viscum album*). Exciting research continues to point to the Maitake mushroom, both as a whole plant and through its extracts, as a powerful anti-cancer weapon.(28) And Carnivora, from the Venus flytrap, seems to have a lot going for it (*see Chapter XIII*).

John Heinerman has detailed how useful anti-cancer extracts were isolated from juniper berries, watercress, chaparral and yarrow at Brigham Young University, Utah; how some anti-cancer activity was shown in the flowers of the *Yucca glaucoma* plant at the University of Wyoming; and even how sunflower extracts were shown in Wyoming lab work to be useful against animal melanoma and leukemia.(29)

Perhaps the most ancient of medicinal herbs known to Western history, garlic, has come into its own for a vast variety of medical reasons, including some specific anti-cancer effects and the isolation from it of a major extract, allicin, which seems to have numerous medical benefits. The same is true for chaparral, an Indian curative from the Southwest prized for numerous purposes (including, through modern research, isolation of an anti-cancer fighter, NDGA, or nordihydroguaiaretic acid) — and which, to nobody's particular surprise, ran afoul of the American FDA in the 1990s.

The pandemic of AIDS — about a quarter of which is comprised of various "forms" of cancer which appear in the presence of a radically depressed immune system — has caused yet a third phase of scrambling for new information on herbs and their extracts which may be immune modulators, anti-carcinogens or antivirals. Increased information on the healing nature of aloe vera, blue-green algae, spirulina, ginseng, and licorice has been in no small part spurred by the drive to find an "AIDS cure."

The US owes a debt of gratitude to the National Cancer Institute's Dr. Jonathan L. Hartwell, who — despite the NCI's predilection for research into toxic compounds (chemotherapy) — as early as 1960 abstracted many years of solid research into North American anti-cancer herbs.

He offered truly vital information on the subject in an orthodox journal.[30]

Thanks primarily to his work, which essentially dwelt on 60 herbs, we know that a powder or liquid application of alfalfa and an oak tree fungus were known to California natives as a general anti-cancer tonic; wild mustard has been used for skin cancer; folklore medicine had it that a poultice of lobelia together with a tea of ginger and soda was useful for breast cancer; that in Pennsylvania of old a tomato juice/alcohol/iodine combination was known to work against liver cancer.

His research, seconded by others, found that "cancer in general" was known to respond to Woodland angelica, burdock, cocklebur, yellow dock, sarsaparilla, dandelions, branches and roots of the elder tree, queen's delight, red clover, sassafras, sycamore, violets (in combination with other plants), and wintergreen.

The fact that so many herbs, plants and combinations thereof were found either by natives or the earlier herb doctors of America to be useful for "cancer in general" (while, indeed, certain decoctions, gels and powders might seem to be targeted for specific accessible tumors, such as those on the skin or lips) is a distant suggestion as to the unitarianism of cancer (*see Chapter IV*) rather than its being several hundred different diseases, as still believed by the majority of American oncologists.

In its unceasing search for the cure for cancer, medical orthodoxy has apparently not taken into consideration the possibility that there may be no single "magic bullet," but possibly many substances having varying degrees of effectiveness against cancer. Stated in simple terms, one side (orthodoxy) says "many diseases, one cure" (or at least one cure for each), while the other side says "one disease, many cures." This is an over-simplification, of course, and the answer may lie somewhere between these two extremes.

All such information originally was empirical — that is, observed — and it would clash with "the scientific method" toward the end of the 19th century, when American medicine took the awesome misstep of trying to become a "science" and needing to "prove" that which was observed.

That a great number of herbs, plants and natural nutrients were somehow useful against cancer was a widely observed phenomenon long before anyone had any real understanding of immune systems let alone antioxidants and phytochemicals. The fact that the "single ingredient" — if there was one — which caused a specific plant to be of value in cancer might not be known caused the rising imperial allopathy of the 19th century to deny the abundance of knowledge gathered through generations of folk medicine.

Some nutrients, such as co-enzyme Q10, basically from animal sources, have produced such favorable anti-cancer effects that they are considered anti-cancer "drugs" in and of themselves.(31) And some products derived from natural sources have been found to be of such general benefit for so many reasons that they could be defined as "natural drugs." Such is the case with DMSO (dimethyl sulfoxide), a byproduct of the newsprint industry (*see Chapter XIII*).

There was of course a far greater reason why American orthodox medicine for the longest time wished to downplay herbs, vitamins and other natural things. It is not the province of this book to delve deeply into it (other writers having done so in considerable detail(32,33) — and that is, natural anti-cancer medicines are unpatentable, cheap, and ubiquitous. There is simply no real profit in dandelion tea or cranberry poultices. The pharmaceutical engine which took over and started driving Western medicine in the late 19th century and throughout the present one became interested in plant-based medicines only to be able to find active ingredients and to manufacture extremely expensive synthetic "analogues" of them to be sold under the guise of "scientific medicine."

Simple greed hence helps explain why so much utterly vital and useful medical knowledge based on herbs and their utility against cancer (and so many other things) was shut out or hidden from public view for so long.

REFERENCES

1. Cameron, Ewan, and Pauling, Linus, *Vitamin C and Cancer.* Menlo Park CA: Pauling Institute of Science and Medicine, 1979.

2. Stone, Irwin, *The Healing Factor: Vitamin C Against Disease.* New York: Grosset and Dunlap, 1972.

3. Riordan, N., *et al.,* "Intravenous ascorbate as a tumor cytotoxic chemotherapeutic agent." *Med. Hypoth.* 44 (3): 205, 1995.

4. Vojdani, A., and Ghoneum, M., "In vivo effects of ascorbic acid on enhancement of human natural killer cell activity." *Nutr. Res.* 13: 753-4, 1993.

5. Goldfarb, R.H., and Herberman, R.B., "Natural killer cell reactivity: regulatory interactions among phorbol ester, interferon, cholera toxin and retinoic acid." *J. Immunol.* 126: 2129, 1981.

6. Dennert, G., and Lotan, R., "Effects of retinoic acid on the immune system: stimulation of T-killer cell induction." *Eur. J. Immunol.* 8: 23, 1978.

7. Dennert, G., *et al.,* "Retinoic acid stimulation of the induction of mouse killer T-cells in allogeneic and synergeneic systems." *J. Natl. Cancer Inst.* 62: 89, 1979.

8. Miscksche, M., *et al.,* "Effect of vitamin A in the treatment of metastatic unresectable squamous cell carcinoma of the lung." *Oncology* 34: 234, 1977.

9. Paganelli, G., *et al.,* "Effect of vitamin A, C, and E supplementation on rectal cell proliferation in patients with colorectal adenomas." *J. Natl. Cancer Inst.* 84: 47-51, 1992.

10. Dartigues, J., *et al.,* "Dietary vitamin A, beta-carotene and risk of epidermoid lung cancer in southwestern France." *Eur. Jour. Epidem.* 6: 261-5, 1990.

11. Gridley, G., *et al.,* "Vitamin supplement use and reduced risk of oral and pharyngeal cancer." *Am. J. Epidem.* 135: 1083-1092, 1992.

12. Bostick, R., *et al.,* "Reduced risk of colon cancer with high intake of vitamin E; The Iowa Women's Health Study." *Canc. Res.* 53: 4230-37, 1993.

13. Benner, S., and Winn, R., *et al.,* "Regression of oral leukoplakia with alpha-tocopherol: a community clinical oncology program chemoprevention study." *J. Nat. Canc. Inst.* 85: 44-47, 1993.

14. Tengerdy, R., "Vitamin E, immune response and disease resistance." In: Diplock, *et al., eds., Vitamin E biochemistry and health implications. Ann. NY Acad. Sci.* 570: 335-44, 1989.

15. Bendich, A., "Antioxidant micronutrients and immune responses." In: Bendich, A., and Chandra, R., *eds., Micronutrients and Immune Functions. Ann. NY Acad. Sci.* 587: 168-180, 1990.

16. Meydani, S., and Tengerdy, R., "Vitamin E and immune response." In: Parker, L., and Fuchs, J., *eds., Vitamin E in Health and Disease.* 4, pp 549-561. New York: Marcel Decker, 1993.

17. Bendich, A., "Antioxidant vitamins and immune responses." In: Chandra, R. (*ed.*), *Nutrition and Immunology,* 125-148. NY: Allan R. Liss, 1988.

18. Finch, J., and Turner, R., "Enhancement of bovine lymphocyte responses: a comparison of selenium and vitamin E supplementation." *Vet. Immunol. Immunopathol.* 23: 245-256, 1980.

19. Jensen, M., *et al.,* "The effect of vitamin E on the cell-mediated immune response in pigs." *J. Vet. Med. Br.* 35: 549-555, 1988.

20. Kowdley, K., *et al.,* "Vitamin E deficiency and impaired cellular immunity related to intestinal fat malabsorption." *Gastroent.* 102: 2139-42, 1992.

21. Vogel, V.J., *American Indian Medicine.* Norman, OK: University of Oklahoma Press, 1970.

22. Hutchens, A.R., *Indian Herbalogy of North America.* Windsor, Canada: Merco, 1973.

23. Boik, J., *Cancer and Natural Medicine.* Princeton, MN: Oregon Medical Press, 1995.

24. Lien, E.J., and Li, W.Y., *Structure-Activity Relationship Analysis of Chinese American Drugs and Related Plants.* Long Beach, CA: Oriental Healing Arts Institute, 1985.

25. Hoxsey, Harry, *You Don't Have to Die.* 1956. Reprinted: Chapala, Mexico: Nature Heals, 1977.

26. Culbert, M.L., *What the Medical Establishment Won't Tell You that Could Save Your Life.* Norfolk, VA: Donning, 1983.

27. Heinerman, J., *The Treatment of Cancer with Herbs.* Orem, UT: BiWorld Publishers, 1984.

28. Nanba, H., "Maitake D-fraction healing and preventing potentials for cancer." *Townsend Letter for Doctors and Patients,* Feb/Mar 1996.

29. Heinerman, *op. cit.*

30. Hartwell J. L., "Plant remedies for cancer." *Cancer Chemother. Reports* 7, 1960.

31. Lockwood, K., *et. al.,* "Partial and complete regression of breast cancer in patients in relation to dosage of coenzyme Q10." *Biochem. and Biophys. Res. Comm.* 199, 1994.

32. Griffin, G.E., *World without Cancer.* Westlake Village, CA: American Media, 1974.

33. Culbert, M. L., *Medical Armageddon.* San Diego CA: C & Communications, 1995.

Chapter IX
LAETRILE (AMYGDALIN, "VITAMIN B17")
Medical Controversy of the Age

A majority of so-called "alternative" cancer clinics, primarily in Mexico, have long used laetrile even while the US cancer establishment, following the "laetrile war" of the 1970s, attempted to write it off as both "highly toxic" and "worthless" — terms which might better be applied to that establishment's own dangerous chemotherapeutic agents.

After years of observing patients using laetrile, also known by its more common generic name of amygdalin or nitriloside, and even as "Vitamin B17," I can say with complete assurance that this compound, especially when used in any rational way, is neither toxic nor worthless.

But neither is it a panacea or cure-all for cancer.

Our own clinic's experience has been that amygdalin or laetrile, given intravenously or orally, has — whatever else — been able to relieve cancer-associated pain rather consistently, leading to the elimination or reduction of pain medication, and that it also enhances the patient's overall well-being.

I have no doubt, after years of observation, that the modern-era laetrile protocols, which involve protein-digesting (proteolytic) enzymes and such major antioxidant vitamins as C and A, exert a direct, anti-cancer benefit while also helping stimulate appetite and energy.

Laetrile is at the heart of the most riveting controversy in modern American medical history. We cannot detail the full story here, since it has been done by many others, particularly including one of the writers (Culbert)**(1)**, but it comes down to this:

Since ancient times, it was known that the black or brown bitter fruit seeds (particularly of apricots, pears, prunes, peaches) and bitter almonds were curative of accessible tumors — and, in overdoses provided for their negative effect, could also function as poisons.

The Egyptians used large amounts of kernels provided to starving prisoners as a poison; a millenium later, the Romans used "bitter almond water" (*aqua amygdalarum amarum*) as a tonic or cure-all.**(2)**

The ancient Sumerians utilized a poultice of nitriloside-rich juniper berries, prune kernels and dried wine dregs for a skin disease which may have been malignant melanoma.**(3)** The ancient Chinese treated tumors with seeds and kernels from nitrilosidic plants and, in this century, have used several species of prunes (the *Prunasae* family containing among the highest levels of natural laetriles) against cancer.**(4)**

The Assyrians utilized various fruit-derived medicines for conditions whose symptoms have been described as "swellings" or "growths" even though the term "cancer" was not used.**(5)**

In the 17th century English herbalist John Gerarde found that an extract of peach kernels was useful for "stoppings of the liver and spleen [and] those who have the Apoplexy."**(6)**

It was during the American Civil War that the value of fruit kernels, primarily of the *Rosaceae* and *Prunasae*, became apparent, with noted Confederate surgeon Dr. Francis Peyre Porcher citing the hydrocyanic acid in peach kernels as the agent primarily responsible for the kernels' medical benefits.**(7)**

In the 19th century, the active principle in the various seeds was determined to be the cyanide-bearing sugar compound amygdalin. Since then, both European and American research found similar compounds (often described as "nitrilosides") in some 1200 edible plants, seeds and grasses. All are considered to be "laetriles," a name which was originally concocted as a brand for a hoped-for non-toxic anticancer drug in the 1920s.

Significant epidemiological data has linked the high consumption of laetrile-bearing (nitrilosidic) foods in well-studied "primitive" human populations with statistically lower rates of cancer in humans as well as in undomesticated animals.**(8)**

In the land of Hunza in the Himalayas, where the apricot and its seed are regularly consumed in large quantities, there has been virtually no cancer in all of the 2000 years of its recorded history. This astounding fact has somehow been omitted from modern-day epidemiology studies.**(9)**

Such respected scientists as the late Dean Burk PhD, a founder of the National Cancer Institute (NCI) and for many years head of its cytochemistry division, believed that the essential non-toxicity of the nitrilosides, their seeming ubiquity in nature, perhaps second only to vitamin C in abundance, and their solubility in water should rightly classify them altogether as a B vitamin — the 17th in order of elucidation, or Vitamin B17.**(10)**

While the cancer establishment in the 1970s vigorously sought to rebut the vitamin argument by claiming that the primary characteristic of a nutrient which makes it a vitamin — namely, a pathological condition arising in its absence — was lacking in the matter of laetrile or Vitamin B17, laetrile proponents begged to differ.

There *is* a pathological condition arising in its absence, and it is cancer. This was the simplistic, if often effective, argument in contending that nitriloside compounds should be treated as foods, nutrients and vitamins, and not as drugs.

Laetrile was to become what the American Cancer Society (ACS) and other elements of the American cancer establishment would call "the political success of a scientific failure," since an amazing 24 states of the USA eventually "decriminalized" its use over the howls of outrage from the ACS, the Food and Drug Administration (FDA) and the American Medical Association (AMA), even when proof of exactly how laetrile "worked" was often lacking.

Even so, several doctors, a recent one being Ohio's Philip Binzel Jr., wrote papers or entire books filled with cases of recoveries or near-recoveries of patients on laetrile-centered anti-cancer treatments, and in state after state more and more doctors came forward to testify that they had found merit in the compound.**(11,12,13)**

The attempted scientific undoing of the laetrile movement occurred in 1980-81, with the NCI-sponsored "laetrile clinical trial," conducted at several American research hospitals, and, as laetrile proponents pointed out, entirely in the hands of anti-laetrile scientists.

A sober rebuttal of the "findings"**(14)** made it clear that, despite the fact that a government-produced product was used in the trial, that agreed-upon protocols were often not followed, and even that some "terminal" patients in the test program who did "too well" were asked to leave it, the small type in the final report did *not* sustain the announced findings as to the "worthlessness" of laetrile.

Indeed, even with a government-produced version of uncertain purity, injectable laetrile led to significant stabilization in either a high plurality or low majority of advanced patients. After the IV program ended and the oral program — not well adhered-to, laetrile proponents would claim — continued there was a descent of most of these already-terminal patients into death. Would this descent have occurred had the IV program not been stopped?

While, from a scientific point of view, the trial raised far more questions than answers, it politically brought the state-to-state drive for laetrile decriminalization to an end, and, for a time, caused a considerable decrease in the use, licit or illicit, of laetrile products, often coming into the US primarily from Mexico but also from Germany, the Caribbean and Asia.

Even so, the "metabolic virus " had been let loose by the laetrile controversy — could a simple food factor actually help prevent cancer? And, if so, following the old medical adage that "that which prevents also cures," couldn't it be true that laetrile, or something like it, could successfully treat cancer?

Just as the laetrile controversy was dying on the nitrilosidic vine, the national furor over vitamin C (thanks primarily to the late Linus Pauling PhD and Ewan Cameron MD in the Vale of Leven, Scotland, trials, followed by a laetrile-like trap trial sponsored in the US) was getting underway. As in the case of laetrile, the vitamin C results raised more questions than answers.

The movement to recognize nutritional therapies as effective against chronic disease in general and cancer in particular was thus jump-started by the political razzle-dazzle of the laetrile movement, the first time a useful but prohibited anti-cancer treatment had "gone political" in the US.

And this was because laetrile proponents had learned lessons from a parallel and earlier era — such useful anti-cancer treatments as Krebiozen, Glyoxylide and the Hoxsey herbals, to name only the major few of a long list of suppressed therapies, all of which had considerable evidence of efficacy for them, had gradually been ground down by a well-oiled coalition of vested interests some have called Cancer Inc. None had "gone political" but laetrile did so. The result was the metabolic revolution in cancer.

On reassessing the "laetrile war" years, it can be said that proponents did not always agree on *how* laetrile was effective against cancer. The primary modern-era pioneer of the compound, the innovative late San Francisco physician, Ernst T. Krebs Sr. MD, had truly believed he had at hand an anti-cancer drug. His biochemist son and a research group believed that the compound worked by the body's creating the "true laetrile compound" (mandelonitrile diglucuronide), which is the result of breaking down natural amygdalin and its conjugation with glucuronic acid to make it non-toxic to the body.

Under this theory, mandelonitrile-glucuronic acid will break down to the primary constituents (benzaldehyde and cyanide) by exploiting the cancer cell's leaky membrane and its ostensibly higher level of the enzyme beta-glucuronidase. Liberation of both poisons within the cancer cell theoretically would provide a one-two punch against both the aerobic and anaerobic processes of malignancy. The original product, injectable amygdalin, hence was described as an essentially non-toxic compound which could be therapeutically effective only against a cancer cell while leaving a normal one untouched.

This sequence of events was probably simplistically overstated by laetrile's proponents while called into question by cancer orthodoxy, and also varied from the presumed route of action of oral laetrile: the conversion of dietary cyanide into the highly useful compound *thiocyanate* by the enzyme rhodanese in the presence of sulfur. Thiocyanate's presumptive attack on cancer is through the release of benzaldehyde, known to attack the *anaerobic* (oxygen-less) condition of a cancer cell.

And, over time, injectable laetrile products did not always live up to advance billing, a point seized upon by the orthodox opposition. Often, inappropriately manufactured IV laetrile turned out to be unstable and would break down to any of a dozen amygdalin-*like* compounds, even though most of them had some benefit. Yet dramatic responses in many cases of cancer were the norm when the liquid product was stable and correct protocols followed.

Later, Japanese research demonstrated anti-cancer effects from the benzaldehyde portion of the compound itself.**(15)**

However, as in the case of aspirin — whose *modus operandi* has not been fully understood over a century of use and whose source of natural derivation is structurally not far distant from the "Vitamin B17" compounds — it was not necessary for doctors to know every biochemical detail of just how laetrile, or any other medication, worked; it was enough to know that laetrile, orally or injectably administered, provided a wide range of benefits, pain relief, stimulation of appetite and energy, sometimes improved blood pressure, and clear evidence of direct anti-cancer benefits.

The controversy over "how laetrile works" straddled the onset of the oxidology revolution (*see Chapter VII*) and it became clear, particularly in 1980 research published by Rutgers University, that, whatever else amygdalin was doing in the body, it was an effective "scavenger" of the most deleterious of the oxygen free radicals, the hydroxyl radical (OH$^{\bullet}$).**(16)**

Since new research continued to show that the way in which cancer spreads, or metastasizes, involves the considerable generation of what some have called reactive oxygen toxic species (ROTS) or simply reactive oxygen species (ROS), beginning with hydrogen peroxide and moving through the "free radical cascade" until hydroxyl radical results, part of laetrile's effectiveness could be seen in a whole new light.

Whatever else, amygdalin and such sister compounds as prunasin, linamarin, dhurrin, lotaustralin and sambunigrin are acting as antioxidants, that is, as scavengers or inhibitors of the toxic oxygen breakdown products which (as ROTS, ROS or free radicals) may attack every major system in the body.

In a way, the laetrile theory — part of which, for North Temperate dwellers, means that folks *should* eat (rather than spit out) black and brown bitter fruit seeds — puts new emphasis on the aphorism that "an apple a day keeps the doctor away."

In more modern parlance, this should be altered to "a whole apple a day, including the seeds, keeps the oncologist at bay."

REFERENCES

1. Culbert, M.L., *Freedom from Cancer.* New York: Pocket Books, 1976.
2. Summa, H.M., "Amygdalin, a physiologically active therapeutic agent in malignancies." Germany: *Krebsgeschehen* 4, 1972.
3. Civil, M., "Prescriptions medicales sumeriennes." France: *Rev.d' Assyriologie* 54, 1960.
4. *Herbal Pharmacology of the People's Republic of China,* cited in Heinerman, John, *The Treatment of Cancer with Herbs.* Orem, UT: Biworld Publishers, 1984.
5. Thompson, R.C., *The Assyrian Herbal.* London: 1924. Cited in Heinerman, *op.cit.*
6. Gerarde, J., *The Herball or Generall Historie of Plantes.* London: 1633. Cited by Heinerman, *op. cit.*
7. Porcher, F.P., *Resources of the Southern Fields and Forests.* Charleston: 1863. Cited by Heinerman, *op. cit.*

8. Krebs, E.T., and Bouziane, N.R., *The Laetriles — Nitrilosides — in the Prevention and Control of Cancer.* Sausalito, CA: The McNaughton Foundation, 1967.

9. Griffin, G.E., *World Without Cancer.* Westlake Village CA: American Media, 1974.

10. Burk, Dean, *A Brief on Foods and Vitamins.* Sausalito, CA: The McNaughton Foundation, 1975.

11. Binzel, P.E., *Alive and Well.* Westlake Village CA: American Media, 1995.

12. Richardson, J.A., *Laetrile Case Histories.* New York: Bantam, 1976.

13. Navarro, M.D., "Laetrile — the Ideal Anti-Cancer Drug?" Manila: *Santo Tomas J. Med.* 10, 1955.

14. *Response of the Committee for Freedom of Choice in Cancer Therapy, Inc. to the National Cancer Institute 'Amygdalin (Laetrile) Clinical Trial.'* Los Altos, CA: CFCCT, Jan. 29, 1982.

15. Tatsumura, T., *et al.,* "4, 6-0-benzylidene-D-glucopyranose (BG) in the treatment of solid malignant tumors." *Br. J. Cancer* 62, 1990.

16. Heikkila, R.E., and Cabbat, F.S., "The prevention of Alloxan-induced diabetes by amygdalin." *Life Sciences* 27, 1980.

Chapter X
PHYTOCHEMICALS
Nature's Chemotherapy

Phytochemicals and phyto-extracts (literally plant chemicals or plant extracts) have been used as medicines throughout history in virtually all cultures. For many centuries knowledge of these materials has been handed down from one generation to the next, a vast body of folk wisdom in which specific plant parts have been used both for specific medical purposes and also as spices for food.

All herbal medicines are derived from plants or plant parts, such as roots, stems, seeds, fruit, leaves, or bark, and each component has its unique medicinal action. Many prescription drugs are derived from these plant substances, and most of these were developed as a result of tracing traditional uses of such natural medicines.

Such phytochemicals, considered non-nutritive since they have no actual food value, have been shown to be useful for a wide variety of human diseases, especially the so-called degenerative diseases such as heart disease and cancer. They apparently act not only to prevent cancer but to help the body attack cancer in a number of ways.(1)

It is ironic that, just as the metabolic revolution in medicine was beginning to get the American public acquainted with vitamins, minerals and other natural nutrients as useful against cancer and other chronic diseases, the area of phytochemicals opened up and took on a life of its own.

By mid-decade, information from biochemistry and epidemiology was pouring in from all sides that not only were the known war-horse vitamins, minerals and related nutrients being demonstrated as anti-chronic disease factors, but a whole host of other plant-based chemicals are, too.

The laetrile controversy (*see Chapter IX*), as we have seen, was paralleled by the announcement that certain compounds similar in structure to amygdalin and its cousins — though allegedly not acting on the same biochemical principles as the same — were useful against cancer. These were generally referred to as *isothiocyanates* — "equal-sulfur-cyanic-acid-related compounds" — and they were said to be widespread in nature.

Interestingly, various of the plant families in which the "B17" nitrilosides are found, including the *Brassica* and *Cruciferae*, contain isothiocyanates or isothiocyanate-similar phytochemicals, which would make the case for their consumption for anti-cancer effects whether one were seeking "Vitamin B17" or not:

Johns Hopkins University research found that some of these phytochemicals inhibit so-called "phase 1" enzymes, which are believed to activate cancer-causing chemicals which initiate the malignant process through damage to cellular DNA. Others are thought to induce "phase 2" enzymes, which at least indirectly check malignancy through the detoxification process.(2)

Related to the isothiocyanates, *sulfuraphane* (from broccoli) and the *indoles* (particularly indole-3-carbinol, from cauliflower, cabbage and broccoli) are involved in blocking the cancer-causing (carcinogenesis) process. Indoles have been shown experimentally to exert a preventive effect against cancers of the breast, colon and stomach, as well as to have a protective effect against the harmful effects of radiation.(3)

Perhaps the greatest amount of phytochemical attention has focused on the soy foods, long a staple in Oriental diets. The *isoflavones* from such foods have been shown to stop the growth of cancer cells *in vitro* and to reduce breast cancer risk in rats.

Isoflavones are chemically similar to the estrogens, but with only a small fraction of the hormonal potency. They are able to compete with estrogen at "receptor sites," preventing the estrogen from activating breast cancer cells, thus acting in much the same way as the drug Tamoxifen. Orientals whose diet is rich in isoflavones have a very low incidence of breast cancer. These plant chemicals are also effective against many other "types" of cancer, such as prostate, lung and colon.

Related flavonoids (from soy foods, apples and onions) have a broad range of utility. Three of these — *genistein, diadzein,* and *quercetin* — have been associated with anticancer effects in animal breast cancer and, in the case of genistein, to interfere with the capacity of cancers to create their own blood vessels (angiogenesis), a process necessary for the nourishment and therefore the growth of all tumors. Thus genistein is an inhibitor of angiogenesis, similar to the known effects of shark cartilage and likely more effective in inhibiting cancer growth.**(4)**

From the same family, *silymarin,* from artichokes, may function as an antioxidant and seems to protect against experimentally induced skin cancer in animals.

Also functioning as antioxidants are *phenols,* found virtually in all fresh fruits, vegetables and cereal grains. As a group, phenols seem to inhibit mutagenesis — capacity to change form, a preliminary step in malignancy — and carcinogenicity itself. One of the more common phenols, *ellagic acid*, is found in walnuts, strawberries, cranberries and blackberries, among many plants.

Recent research has shown that green and black teas, also staples of the Oriental diet, are effective against tumor formation, probably because of their high degree of phenolic compounds.

Even orange peels and the oils of other citrus fruits, by producing *monoterpenes* such as *D-limonene* and *perillyl alcohol*, have been found useful against experimental tumor systems. And *pectin*, the "cement" of fruit cell walls, has been found in animal tests to help fight prostate and lung cancer.

Tannins, isolated from grapes and wine, may have antioxidant effects against cancer and are part of the reason why conservative wine consumption, other than for those genetically prone to develop alcoholism or who are under diabetic or yeast treatments, is increasingly recommended for good health.

Phytate is a plant-derived iron-binding substance thought to be active in the prevention of free radical formation, a factor in the development of cancer cells.

Phytochemicals of one kind or another undoubtedly play roles in what one of the writers (Culbert, together with researcher D.I. Camino) called "the condiment surprise" in 1994.

Bradford Research Institute (BRI) research found an unexpected role for spices, condiments and seasonings in cancer prevention and noted that such elements are often lacking in such modern manufactured food composites as "TV dinners."

Scanning world dietary information, BRI researchers found that many of the seasonings used by peoples around the world are known to have some cancer-blocking effects, particularly through activation of the liver detoxification apparatus called the MFO, or mixed-function oxidase system.**(5)**

Hence, there is now an anti-cancer rationale for ingesting celery seeds, caraway seeds, rosemary, nutmeg, cloves, parsley, mustard, lemon grass, gulanga root, curry, betel leaves and ginger.

And a reason why various products combining several phytochemicals began appearing in the mid-1990s as potent anti-cancer fighters isolated from both common and not-so-common foods, yet none of which were classified as vitamins but often as "non-nutritive food factors."

There is little wonder that National Cancer Institute (NCI) consultant Mark Messina has called phytochemicals "absolutely the hottest area in nutrition — they will be the vitamins and minerals of the 21st century."(6)

And their utility, of course, is not limited strictly to cancer, but to the sum total of nutritional factors involved in promoting health and preventing chronic disease.

The tragedy has long been that so few research funds have been available to look extensively into Mother Nature's vast pharmacopeia to find and prove the thousands of useful compounds that abound therein, while billions have gone into developing "synthetic analogues" of the same as well as wholly manufactured (usually, from petrochemicals) synthetic drugs.

I have found, in alignment with early research, that the isoflavones in particular seem to be unusually effective against the so-called hormone-dependent cancers, such as breast and prostate.

I recommend that patients consume abundant quantities of cabbage, kohlrabi, cauliflower, Brussels sprouts and the omnipresent broccoli not only because of so many already recognized vitamins and minerals in them but also because they contain so many of the ever-lengthening list of phytochemicals.

REFERENCES

1. Steinmetz, K., and Potter, J., "Vegetables, fruit and cancer. *Cancer Causes and Control.* 2: 325-357 (Part I), 2: 427-442 (Part II), 1991.
2. Marwick, Charles, "Learning how phytochemicals help fight disease." *J. Am. Med. Assn.* 274, Nov. 1, 1995.
3. Albert, P.N., *J. Ethnopharmacol.* 1983; Stoesand, G.S., 1988; and Michnovicz, J.J., *J. Natl. Cancer Inst.* 1990.

4. Fotsis, T., *et al.,* "Genistein, a dietary-derived inhibitor of *in vitro* angiogenesis." *Proc. Natl. Acad. Sci. USA* 90: 1993.

5. Culbert, M.L., and Camino, D.I., *Nutritional Factors in the Prevention and Management of Cancer.* San Diego, CA: C and C Communications, 1995.

6. At the American Institute for Cancer Research Convention, Washington DC, October 1995.

Chapter XI
UKRAIN AND GREATER CELANDINE
Hope from a 3,500-year-old Herb

Ukrain, derived from *Chelidonium majus,* one of the most ancient herbs known to man, has shown powerful immune-stimulating effects in patients with a variety of cancers.(1)

This refined extract, combined with another non-toxic substance, has the ability to inhibit cancer growth selectively while not only doing no harm but actually fortifying the body's defense system.(2)

In the past few years, a number of clinical studies have demonstrated that Ukrain is capable of improving the general conditions and prolonging the lives of terminal cancer patients by boosting their immune systems and inhibiting tumor growth.(3)

With all of these unique attributes, one would think that Ukrain would have been embraced by the American cancer establishment.

After all, it went through a large part of the National Cancer Institute (NCI) testing procedures in 1992 and was found effective in a stunning 18 of 23 "cell lines" against which it was tested. Its greatest efficacy, even at the NCI, was against small-cell lung cancer, melanoma, colon, ovarian, non-small cell lung, and cancers of the central nervous system — that is, some of the top killer cancers.(4)

Besides, it is essentially non-toxic, distancing it, even as a drug, from the toxic chemotherapeutic compounds favored by the American medical establishment.

Instead of creating great excitement at the NCI, this highly promising naturally derived material was apparently shelved. Could this be due to the fact that this herbal product — call it a drug if you must — was developed in Europe, not in the US, and may not be patentable in this country?

As of summer 1996, a check with the NCI found Ukrain "not in the computer" and thus assumed — as verified by the FDA — to be "an illegal new drug" if promoted in the USA as a cancer treatment.(5) Of course, Americans were known to be ordering the product from

Europe and it was available for general use in at least one "alternative" clinic in Mexico.

While researched and tested in Austria and elsewhere in Europe for some two decades, where notable successes have been achieved, Ukrain remains "unapproved" in the USA.

My own experience with this injectable drug — a semisynthetic derivative of the ancient herb known as greater celandine (*Chelidonium majus*) complexed with thiophosphoric acid — sustains what the relatively extensive research shows: some kind of efficacy against virtually all cancers with the possible exception of leukemias.

Ukrain's utility in the anti-cancer arena is not limited to its demonstrated ability to interfere with cancer cell division (mitosis); it also is known to elevate that portion of the immune system, the natural killer (NK) cells, which are essential both to the body's defense against malignant conditions and regulation of T-cells. These features make it a potential anti-AIDS treatment as well.**(6,7)**

None of this should amaze any student of natural medicines. Greater celandine, from the poppy family, has been known to generations of folk healers, herbalists and even homeopaths for a broad range of immune-boosting and anti-cancer, liver-cleansing and many other effects.

It was Austrian doctors, originally from the Ukraine (hence the name as spelled in German), who began developing and testing the semisynthetic derivative some two decades ago, even though other research was done on other useful alkaloids from this truly amazing herb.

The Ukrain story is symptomatic of what is wrong with the American FDA drug-approval process.

Here we have a foreign-developed, foreign-tested drug with substantial *in vitro*, animal and clinical (that is, live human) research behind it, generally available to much of the world, but yet not cleared through the FDA drug-approval process which, depending on who is counting and which elements are involved, may take anywhere from $250 to $350 million in costs and many years in development time.**(8)**

Additionally, the raw material from which the drug — and in the case of greater celandine, several drugs — is derived has been well-known and easily available as a wild herb for thousands of years.

It is true that Ukrain's developers, following the usual allopathic methods and standards, have sought to manufacture, license and control a "drug" in the precise definition of the word, and that the funds spent on the drug so far deal with a specific product (Ukrain) rather than with all aspects of the herb itself.

The problem with "testing herbs" in the Western world is that every herb is a composite of several dozen to several hundred or more possibly useful compounds, and these may be concentrated in their tops, roots, stems, leaves or other parts.

Discovering exactly which properties in which parts of which herbs are useful requires an enormous outlay of funds, costs which are prohibitive unless the final extract or ingredient is to be altered in some proprietary way to constitute a synthetic and patentable new compound. When this is the goal, the investment in research time and money is expected to pay off in terms of at least temporary monopolistic control over a product legally entered into the market.

The more we know about Ukrain, the product, and about greater celandine (*Chelidonium majus*), its herb of origin, the better they both look, but of course the finished injectable product (Ukrain) is far more expensive than the herb in its natural state. So more can be specifically stated about specific uses of the drug than of the herb.

Early results from its use at a Mexican clinic showed responses against cancer, including Kaposi's sarcoma, a common (and deadly) feature of AIDS.(9)

Although celandine-based medications have been known in Europe and Asia for the better part of four millenia, it was British apothecary/herbologist Nicholas Culpeper who, in the 17th century, did much to explain, along with herbalist W.J. Simmonite, the nature and uses of the plant.

Culpeper wrote that the herb could be made into an oil ointment "to anoint your poor eyes with" and that "the juice . . . rubbed often on warts will take them away . . . the juice of decoction of the herb gargled between the teeth that ache, easeth the pain."(10)

Culpeper and Simmonite added that greater celandine "grows by old walls, hedges, and untilled places. It has large leaves and yellow flowers . . . It is an herb of the Sun in Leo, and should be gathered when the Sun is in Leo and the Moon in Aries, applying to a trine of Sol. The juice takes off warts, and being dropped in the eye heals sore eyes, helps ringworms, ascorbic eruptions, mercurial sores, and bad legs."(11)

Going into the twentieth century, greater celandine was described as a purgative, caustic and cholagogue with the whole herb and its raw juice being used, even though the most modern research has isolated a majority of the useful alkaloids from roots. A 20th-century accounting of *Chelidonium majus* found that its "raw juice has been used for eczema, ringworm, athlete's foot, warts, and malignant tumors of the skin" as well as for gallstones.**(12)**

Japanese research in 1989 showed that greater celandine, among other traditional (Chinese) herbs, was useful in the treatment of squamous cell carcinoma of the esophagus and that, in general, "the antitumor action of [these] herbs is thought to be brought about by the activation of an immunological rejection mechanism."**(13)**

During the outbreak of the AIDS pandemic, more attention than ever before was focused on natural immune system regulators, and by the early 1980s it was suggested that a bitter tea made from the leaves of the greater celandine exerted some kind of immune stimulation in immunologically compromised patients.

Now that the product Ukrain has been shown to have a regulatory effect on the T-lymphocytes, of key importance in AIDS, in addition to the known property of greater celandine to have a stimulating effect on NK cell activity, it would seem that in this herb and its derivatives we have an ideal immune booster which, unlike the synthetic proteins trumpeted by the medical establishment as the "only" way to stimulate immunity, is essentially non-toxic.

There now are sublingual and oral preparations of concentrated greater celandine which patients are taking for general reasons of good health.

As is the case with virtually all the useful herbs and their derivatives, Ukrain may have even more than immune-regulating and direct anti-cancer capabilities.

Research in 1993 showed that Ukrain "may be useful not only for cytostatic therapy in cancer patients but also in diseases associated with antioxidant insufficiency, e.g., peritonitis and infection complications in cancer patients."**(14)**

The same year, other research suggested Ukrain was also beneficial as an anti-influenza remedy.**(15)**

Also exciting is recent Russian research which showed that greater celandine, tested along with several berries, might be playing a role in inducing resistance to experimental infection by tick-borne encephalitis virus (and, by implication, resistance to other viruses as well.)**(16)**

A survey of existing greater celandine medical literature published in Czechoslovakia in 1995 found that some 30 isoquinolone alkaloids had been isolated from the plant and that the two dominant ones are chelidonium and coptisine.**(17)**

It would seem that the Ukrain/greater celandine scientific story is just beginning.

REFERENCES

1. Nowicky, J.W., "New immuno-stimulating anti-cancer preparation: Ukrain." In: *Proc.* 13th Intl. Cong. Chemother., Vienna, 28, 1983.
2. Nowicky, J.W., *et al.,* "Ukrain as both anti-cancer and immunoregulatory agent." *Drugs Exp. Clin. Res. XVIII (Suppl), 1992.*
3. Lohninger, A. and Hamler, F., "*Chelidonium majus L.* (Ukrain) in the treatment of cancer patients." *Drugs Exp. Clin. Res. XVIII (Suppl), 1992.*
4. Nowicky, J.W., *et al.,* "Cytostatic and cytotoxic effects of Ukrain on malignant cells." Abst. 977, 8th Medit. Cong. Chemother., Athens, 1992.
5. Personal communication, M. L. Culbert, July 1996.
6. Nowicky, J.W. , *et al.,* "Ukrain and natural killer cells." 18th Intl. Cong. Chemother., Stockholm, 1993.
7. Nowicky, J.W., *et al.,* "Evaluation of thiophosphoric acid alkaloid derivatives from *Chelidonium majus L.* ('Ukrain') as an immunostimulant in patients with various carcinomas." Vienna: *Drugs Exp. Clin. Res.* 17, 1991.
8. Culbert, M.L., *Medical Armageddon.* San Diego, CA: C & C Communications, 1995.
9. Culbert, M.L., "Ukrain." Publication of American Biologics-Mexico SA Medical Center, Tijuana, Mexico, and Bradford Research Institute, Chula Vista, CA, 1995.
10. Griggs, Barbara, *Green Pharmacy.* New York: Viking, 1981.
11. *The Simmonite-Culpeper Herbal Remedies.* New York: Award Books, 1957.
12. Carse, Mary, *Herbs of the Earth.* Hinesburg TN: Upper Access, 1989.
13. Xian, M.S., *et al.,* "Efficacy of traditional Chinese herbs on squamous cell carcinoma of the esophagus: histopathological analysis of 240 cases." Japan: *Acta Med. Okayama* 43, 1989.
14. Voltchek, I.V., *et al.,* "Some immunohematological effects of Ukrain." 18th Intl. Cong. Chemother., Stockholm, 1993.
15. Potopalsky, A.L., and Nowicky, J.W., "Semisynthetic antitumor alkaloid derivatives as antiviral and potential anti-HIV preparations." *Antivir. Res.* 20 (Suppl.), Abst. 57, 1993.
16. Fokima, G.I., *et al.,* "The antiviral action of medicinal plant extracts in experimental tick-borne encephalitis." Russia: *Vopr. Virusol* 38, 1993.
17. Taborska, E., *et al.,* "The greater celandine (*Chelidonium majus L.*) — a review of contemporary knowledge." Czech Republic: *Ceska Slov. Farm.* 44, 1995.

Chapter XII
ENZYMES
The Keys to Life

It is amazing to many of us in the alternative camp how little importance Cancer Inc. has given to the role of enzymes in the management of cancer.

These powerfully active natural chemicals are protein-mineral complexes which occur in all living things and make possible virtually all of the many biochemical reactions in the body. They are indispensable to life and to good health.

Whenever there is a significant reduction in the presence or the availability of enzymes, disease and degeneration begin.

These keys to life can be roughly divided into three types: those derived from food, digestive enzymes, and metabolic enzymes.

Food enzymes are abundantly present in all uncooked vegetables, fruits, and grains. They assist in the breakdown of the food in which they are present and also perform other useful functions in the body. Food processing commonly employed today destroys nearly all of the enzymes normally present in foods. Whatever enzymes may remain after processing at the factory are finished off at home on the range.

Cooking by whatever means, except for very light steaming, will completely destroy all enzymes in food — even the foods that were healthy to start with.

Destroying the enzymes in food places an extra burden on the second group, the digestive enzymes. These are normally made by the pancreas, which produces a specific digestive enzyme for the breakdown and assimilation of each type of food we consume — lipase for fats, amylase for carbohydrates or sugars, and proteases for different types of protein.

Metabolic enzymes make up the third and most abundant group of enzymes in the body, and these function within the cell to regulate such activity as detoxification, oxygen utilization and energy production, along with a multitude of life-sustaining and disease-fighting functions.

There are over 3000 enzyme systems at work in the body. Performing a vast number of functions, these indispensable substances hold the keys to life. They assist greatly in the rebuilding of all tissues in the body by breaking down ingested protein into its component amino acids which the body uses as building blocks for repair and rejuvenation. They attack waste materials in the blood and in the tissues, converting them into a form that can be readily eliminated, thereby acting as blood purifiers.

The immune system depends heavily upon enzymes for all of its functions. To enumerate all of the actions of enzymes in detail would take several volumes and need not be elaborated upon in this small book. Suffice it to say that they are essential to the performance of every function of every organ system in our bodies.

Many white blood cells produce and utilize enzymes as a necessary part of their function. Front-line soldiers of the white cell army, called macrophages, discussed elsewhere in this book (*see Chapter VI*), are indispensable fighters of the cellular part of the immune system. They are the "cleanup crew" or "sanitation department" of the body.

Literally "big eaters," these macrophages permeate every tissue in the body, seeking out, attacking, surrounding, ingesting, and digesting, *by enzyme activity,* all foreign materials — toxins from outside and inside the body, dead or dying cells, degenerating cells, and of, course, cancer cells.

Needless to say, these warriors are absolutely essential in protecting the body from cancer as well as in fighting cancer once it has secured a foothold. Great care must be exercised to protect these hungry macrophages lest toxic residues, microorganisms and abnormal cells accumulate in the tissues, blood and lymph, leading to degenerative disease, including cancer.

A myriad of environmental toxins, stress, poor dietary habits, drugs (especially chemotherapeutic agents) all have inhibiting effects on these important fighters and their enzymatic activity.[1]

Another cancer-fighter, the T-lymphocyte, more specifically the killer T-cell, attacks cancer cells in a similar manner, utilizing enzymes in its ability to dissolve and digest tumor cells (*see Chapter VI*). As we have seen, these fighters are part of a highly integrated system capable of recognizing cancer cells, then attacking and destroying them. This information is extensively utilized by alternative care physicians, such as myself, in designing an effective program to combat cancer or any disease, such as AIDS, which has immune deficiency as its principal feature.

Other enzymes, particularly the proteolytic enzymes from the pancreas, have the unique ability to break down the muco-protein coating which encases all malignant tumors and protects cancer cells from attack by the body's immune system.

Enzymes also protect the body against cancer — particularly metastatic or spreading cancer — in other ways.

Pre-cancer cells become attached to body tissues by means of fibrin, a protein component necessary for blood clotting. Enyzmes digest away the fibrin, preventing the attachment of pre-cancerous and cancerous cells to body tissues, thus releasing these abnormal cells into the circulating blood where they are normally destroyed by the fighters described above.

Research has shown that enzymes — in this case, bromelain, a protein-digesting vegetable enzyme — have the power to transform cancer cells to normal cells. This and other evidence seems to indicate that — in addition to their many other attributes — enzymes may have a directly normalizing effect on cancer cells.[1]

Enzymes also have an activating effect on the immune system and are believed to be an integral part of that system. Studies have shown that cancer is associated with severe deficiencies of many enzymes.

This knowledge is not new.

A century ago, Scottish embryologist John Beard (*see Chapter IX*), in spite of having little knowledge of enzymes, discovered that by taking pancreas tissue from young animals he could extract a liquid which was effective in causing tumor reduction.

Practicing in England, Dr. Beard would inject his pancreatic extract either directly into accessible tumors or into the muscle or vein of the patient. Even some advanced cancers considered to be incurable were made to completely disappear. He was able to help or apparently cure over half of his patients, most with advanced cancers, a far cry from today's dismal statistics.[2]

His was a crude preparation, containing impurities and foreign proteins which produced some allergic reactions. For this he was roundly criticized and attacked by his peers in the medical profession, not unlike organized medicine's attacks today on the innovative physician.

His attackers tried to "put him out of business" by discrediting him, pointing to the adverse reactions and to the patients who died despite his treatment. This also reminds us of the prevailing bias among mainstream physicians today — namely, that it is acceptable for a cancer patient to die while under conventional treatment (or because of it), but it is definitely *not* tolerable for this to happen while a patient is under alternative care.

Because there arose such a demand for Dr. Beard's pancreatic enzyme preparation, English physicians were hounded by their cancer patients to be treated with this miraculous substance. Consequently, attempts were made to duplicate the material, pharmacists obtaining pancreatic juice from local slaughterhouses.

The trouble was, the pancreases were taken from older animals with far less enzymatic activity than the younger animals which Beard had made sure were the source of his material.

The other factor which rendered the attempted duplication totally ineffective was the passage of time. Enzymes have a relatively short "shelf life," being "live" substances and remaining active only for a matter of hours after removal from the animal.

Beard had been careful to use only freshly removed pancreases for his material. Thus, the obtaining of material by other physicians through "normal channels," i.e. slaughterhouses, pharmacists, couriers, etc., resulted in enough delay that the enzymes were rendered completely useless.

Since Dr. Beard's colleagues had no success with their inactive enzyme material, the concept and method of treatment sadly fell into disrepute and into obscurity. Fortunately, in 1907 Beard wrote a book about his experiences in treating cancer patients and his hypothesis of the causation of cancer, now known as the "trophoblast" theory, so his work was not completely lost to posterity (*see Chapter IV*).

However, for nearly 50 years there was no significant activity in the area of enzymes and cancer, Beard's work having been forgotten, and consensus medicine of the day having returned to its certainty that enzymes could not have anything to do with cancer, much less anything to do with curing it.

Next on the enzyme scene was Dr. Max Wolf, a professor at Columbia University, New York. Dr. Wolf had developed an interest in enzymes and cancer and had written to all of the medical libraries in the US and much of the Western world seeking information on the subject.

Reading virtually everything that had ever been written about the subject up to that time, Wolf became probably the world's leading authority on enzymes and their relationship to cancer. One of the books he managed to locate and read was John Beard's book, of which there were then precious few remaining.

Working at his research laboratory at Columbia in the 1950s, Wolf designed a complicated and extensive study of the effect of enzymes on cancer cells.**(4,5)** Thousands of cell cultures were prepared with normal cells and cancer cells living and growing together. Each of these cultures was then treated with a particular enzyme or combination of enzymes to determine which was most effective in killing cancer cells while preserving normal ones.

A wide range of enzymes and combinations was tested in this way to establish the most potent combination which would safely avoid damaging normal cells. Because of Wolf's connections in Germany (and because of the inhibiting presence of the American FDA), clinical work was carried out in that country using the final formula on human cancer victims with highly favorable results.

This particular mixture of enzymes survives to this day as Wobe-Mugos — the "Wobe" part being derived from the names Wolf and Benitez (Wolf's partner in all of this work) — which has been used to treat tens of thousands of cancer patients in Germany over approximately the last 30 years. This material, along with a companion product called Wobenzyme, also has also been used in the US by a few physicians, including myself, as well as in several Mexican clinics.

Also available from Germany is an injectable preparation of Wobe-Mugos enzymes, which I have found quite useful in treating accumulations of fluid in the chest, called pleural effusions, when these accumulations are due to cancer. This has been done in Germany for many years with consistent success. Collections of abdominal fluid, called ascites, can be treated in like manner. In addition, any tumor which is accessible by needle may be treated with this material.

These and other similar enzyme products have a wide application in medicine, being effective against many inflammatory conditions — arthritis, autoimmune diseases, injuries, blood clots, and phlebitis, to name a few — as well as against cancer.

I consider enzymes to be indispensable in the management and control of cancer. If I were to be limited to a single nutritional substance in this management, it would probably be enzymes.

To illustrate the importance of enzymes and to show why their decrease or disturbance represents such a prevalent problem in Western society, I would indulge the reader in a brief lesson in anatomy and physiology.

Herbivorous animals (non-cheating vegetarians) have an extra pouch above the stomach which has the purpose of carrying out pre-digestion. As we have seen, raw plant foods contain their own enzymes, and the pre-stomach sac in the animal allows the food to be pre-digested by its own enzymes, along with enzymes in the saliva, before passing on to gastric or stomach digestion. (*See figure A next page.*)

Not well known is the fact that humans have similar equipment for two-stage digestion. Dr. Edward Howell, among others, has done research demonstrating that the human stomach is, physiologically, actually two stomachs, each performing a distinctly separate function. The upper stomach, called the cardiac portion (because of its location beneath the heart, not because it has anything directly to do with the heart), acts as a "storage bag," with none of the peristaltic action (churning) such as that which is present throughout the remainder of the digestive tract.

This portion of the stomach has few, if any, of the glands that secrete hydrochloric acid and enzymes so prevalent in the lower portion of the stomach. This relatively inert bag at the human stomach's upper end corresponds to what Howell calls the food-enzyme stomach in animals, the purpose of which is to allow enzyme-containing foods and salivary enzymes to pre-digest food, preparing it for gastric digestion.(3)

By eating enzyme-poor foods, cooking or processing out what few enzymes remain in food, then eating too much of this, it is easy to see that we of the Western world have under-used our enzyme-food stomachs and placed an extra burden on the remainder of the digestive apparatus.

In the lower or pyloric portion of the stomach, food is more actively broken down by hydrochloric acid, pepsin, and other gastric enzymes. This part of the stomach has very active peristaltic movement in contrast with the relatively quiescent upper part.

Now overburdened by inadequately digested food, the pyloric stomach then passes this burden on to the duodenum or first part of the small intestine, where enzymes from the pancreas try to deal with the bad hand they have been dealt.

Figure A

DIAGRAMMATIC REPRESENTATIONS OF
FOOD-ENZYME STOMACHS

In animals and humans alike, food-enzyme stomachs are always the first stop stations of food in its journey through the digestive tract. In addition to those listed below, numerous species of rodents, monkeys, and bats have cheek pouches and hip pouches to keep food moist and warm so that its food enzymes can perform predigestion.

Food-Enzyme Stomachs Illustrated as Squares in the Following

HUMAN

In humans, the cardiac portion is the food-enzyme stomach.

CHICKEN

In seed-eating birds such as the chicken and the pigeon, the crop is the food-enzyme stomach.

COW

In ruminative animals such as the cow and the sheep, there are three food-enzyme stomachs:

    1st – Rumen
    2nd – Reticulum
    3rd – Omasum

WHALE

In Cetacea such as the dolphin and whale, the 1st stomach is the food-enzyme stomach.

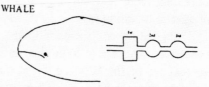

Gray's Anatomy cites the authority Walter B. Cannon who demonstrated that the human stomach "consists of two parts physiologically distinct." *Gray's Anatomy* states: "The cardiac portion of the stomach is a food reservoir in which salivary digestion continues; the pyloric portion is the seat of active gastric digestion. There are no peristaltic waves in the cardiac portion." Predigestion by exogenous (outside) enzymes is widespread in nature. Our enzyme potential has other and more useful and taxing work to do than merely making endogenous digestive enzymes to digest food.

Note: This diagram and accompanying text are taken from Enzyme Nutrition~The Food-Enzyme Concept by Dr. Edward Howell, pp.109-110.

Unwholesome meal after unwholesome meal, year after year, takes a profound toll on the enzyme "pool," the total enzymes available in the intestinal tract and elsewhere.

Like being repeatedly overdrawn at the bank, eventually something bad happens. Not only bad dietary habits but aging further depletes our store of enzymes, contributing to the perpetual withdrawal problem.

It is thus exceedingly important to keep putting "money in the bank" in the form of food enzymes from uncooked vegetables, fruits, grains, sprouts, digestive enzymes and food enzyme supplements.

And this includes supplements to help compensate for the body's store of decreased or missing "antioxidant" enzymes (*see Chapter VII*), which also have a role to play in cancer.

Studies have shown that in patients with pancreatic cancer and post-surgical breast cancer treated with enzymes, survival rates were significantly better than for those not treated with enzymes.(6)

It is my carefully considered opinion that a chronic deficiency of total enzymes available to the body is a major factor contributing to the development of cancer and other degenerative diseases, and that enyzmes from both animal and vegetable sources have a definite place in the management and treatment of the cancer patient.

REFERENCES

1. Maurer, H. *et al.,* "Bromelain induces the differentiation of leukemia cells in vitro: an explanation for its cytostatic effects?" *Planta Med.* 377-81, 1986.

2. Beard, J., *Enzyme Therapy of Cancer.* In Wolf, M. (Hrsg), Vienna: Maudrich-Verlag, 1971.

3. Howell, E., *Enzyme Nutrition — The Food Enzyme Concept.* Wayne NJ: Avery Publishing, 1985.

4. Wolf, M.; Ransberger, K., *Enzyme Therapy.* Vienna, Maudrich-Verlag, 1970.

5. Lopez, D., *et al., Enzymes — The Fountain of Life.* Neville Press, 1994.

6. Boit, J., "Digestive Enzymes." in: *Cancer and Natural Medicine: A Textbook of Basic Science and Clinical Research,* pp 165-6. Princeton, MN: Oregon Medical Press, 1995

Chapter XIII
NEW MODALITIES
The Cancer Calamity Spurs Some Intriguing Discoveries

Due to the seeming incurability by conventional means of most advanced cancers and the dismal track record in this country of the alliance of vested interests and ideas we generally call Cancer Inc., malignancy has always been a magnet for con men and opportunists — a fact not lost on today's "quackbusters."

Yet the nature of the calamity is such that it has also generated new approaches and techniques, some highly useful, others dubious, and some for which the jury is still out.

By no means have all of these come from "unconventional" sources even though they seem to be unconventional themselves.

They are innovative techniques and ideas which, over the course of time, are tending to prove to be of at least some benefit. It is not the province of this book to detail each and every "alternative" approach but rather to concentrate on the main ones and summarize the others.

The use of such oxidative agents as hydrogen peroxide and ozone is, for example, neither from "holistic" origins nor is it new (*see Chapter VII*).

The discovery of multiple benefits from *germanium* and *co-enzyme Q10* made these two agents virtual household words by the 1990s, and with good reason, for their application has led to a wealth of healthful uses, including activity against cancer.

Since Kazuhiko Asai began researching the sesquioxide compounds of germanium now better known as GE-132 and calling the same a "medical godsend,"(1) significant research has found anti-cancer and immune-stimulating properties in this mineral,(2,3,4) so much so that some cancer patients believe its high-dose oral supplementation has been the most important element in their seeming recovery from advanced cancer.(5)

The ongoing interest in germanium is parenthetically a rationale, among others, for the consumption of garlic and ginseng, which are readily available food sources of it.

Co-enzyme Q10, one of the compounds classed as ubiquinones, while long known in Japan as a heart disease remedy and as a useful antioxidant with evidence of anti-cancer effects in animals, particularly came into its own in 1994 thanks to Danish research.

As part of a general protocol involving antioxidants against "high-risk" breast cancer, patients treated with high-dose CoQ10 (300 mg. or 390 mg. daily) either saw total or residual tumor destruction with this agent alone.(8)

As we note elsewhere, a common herb used for almost four thousand years is the basis of the useful drug Ukrain against many "forms" of cancer (*see Chapter XI*).

Another plant-derived substance which has received enthusiastic attention among metabolic physicians is *Carnivora,* a unique substance derived from the Venus flytrap, a carnivorous plant, by Germany's Dr. Helmut Keller.(9)

It has also been given a boost over the years by integrative German physician Hans Nieper MD, and has frequently been used in Mexican alternative cancer clinics. It is among innovative modalities developed and studied by a number of individuals often thought of as at least close to the scientific and medical mainstream.

To hear or read from Carnivora's ever-growing population of enthusiasts, this extract of *Dionaea muscipula,* provided as Carnivorain (for intravenous and intramuscular injection) and as drops for oral and inhalation use, is a "cure" for everything from cancer to AIDS.(10,11)

While controlled studies are hard to come by, the anecdotal evidence is certainly impressive.

Veteran medical journalist Morton Walker found that between 1981 and 1991 some 2,000 persons had been treated with the Venus flytrap product.(12) It has been used at least adjunctively, according to Carnivora's growing underground, even by former President and Mrs. Ronald Reagan as well as the late actor Yul Brynner, who was also known to have used laetrile at some point during his cancer therapy.

There are several anecdotal cases of clearance of HIV, the alleged "AIDS virus," from the blood of AIDS and pre-AIDS patients and notable increases in their immune responses.

Indeed, Carnivora's primary action may be due to the immune-stimulating activity of its primary ingredient, plumbagin (hydroplumbagin-4-0-beta-glucopyranoside).(13)

Carnivora chronicler Dr. Walker has made this observation of Dr. Keller's treatment:

"Yes, Dr. med. Helmut Keller is the discoverer of a correction for cancer, AIDS, and other pathologies. (Dr. Keller has prevailed upon me to refrain from calling it a 'cure' although I believe it comes closer to curing cancer and AIDS than anything else ever uncovered by members of the medical community). The world should be apprised of the therapeutic effects of this treatment. . . "(14)

It remains one of so many natural products continually ignored by the American medical establishment and its Cancer Inc. subdivision which, as we see throughout this book, tends to turn its back on those things which are (a) natural, (b) unpatentable, (c) inexpensive and (d) often resulting from foreign research.

It does not take an expert in murine biology to smell a rat here.

SHARK AND BOVINE CARTILAGE — GATHERING THE EVIDENCE

At this writing, the utilization of cartilage against cancer (and other conditions) is boiling on two fronts: first, as a modality in and of itself, and, second, as a controversy pitting champions of shark-derived cartilage vs. those of bovine-derived material.

The latter includes, as prime players, William Lane PhD (whose book *Sharks Don't Get Cancer(15)* made the use of shark cartilage against malignancy an international issue of broad public interest) and John F. Prudden MD, usually thought of as the father of cartilage therapy.

Entering from stage left was the Cuban government, which, in research in the early 1990s, cautiously confirmed some of the claims made for shark cartilage as suggested by Lane, but fell far short of seeing the material as a guaranteed "cancer cure." This is my position with regard to the effectiveness of shark cartilage.

While Drs. Lane and Prudden have continued to fight it out in "alternative" medical journals,(16,17) there is little doubt that orally consumed cartilage from either source and in relatively high doses has both some immune system-modulating properties and something of central importance to the way in which cancer metastasizes, or spreads.

Cartilage seems to contain certain compounds which are actually able to "turn off" the development of new blood vessels which feed tumors. The process of blood vessel proliferation is called angiogenesis, a unique feature of cancer and its metastatic nature. Cancer's ability to wall itself off from normal tissue and to create its own circulatory system are intriguing and frustrating aspects of the disease.

First, animal research showed, and then clinical (human) use, as in Cuba, seemed to confirm, that under the influence of orally consumed shark cartilage tumors shrank as their blood supplies diminished.

Dr. Prudden, as well as independent researchers in the area,(18,19) have indicated that cartilage (shark or bovine) effects on cancer may have far more to do with immune system modulation than with the inhibition of angiogenesis. The controversy remains unresolved, and shark cartilage has received a federal IND (Investigational New Drug) number for human use against prostate cancer and Kaposi's sarcoma.(20)

In the meantime, the use of oral cartilage products constitutes a generally safe, non-toxic method which many doctors have found useful against chronic disease in general.

DMSO — THE CLOSEST THING TO AN ELIXIR

How the chemical dimethyl sulfoxide (DMSO), a byproduct of the newsprint industry (from paper pulp), came to be found useful for a vast range of medical problems, very much including cancer, is a lengthy story of false premises, false starts, medical economics and politics and battles of clashing paradigms.(21)

In essence, DMSO, while first discovered in Russia in 1866, where its ability to dissolve and transport other substances was first noted, did not begin to come into its own until 1948, when its general physiological properties began to emerge. Even so, it was not until Stanley Jacob MD, an assistant professor of surgery at the University of Oregon Medical School, became interested in the paper pulp byproduct that DMSO took off on a long and zig-zagging medical, scientific and bureaucratic course.

Dr. Jacob suffered years of persecution, defamation and financial hardship, nearly losing his professorship, before more or less resolving the matter with a successful lawsuit against the FDA.

Ultimately, DMSO would be found to have an impressive range of properties (solvent, transporter agent, antioxidant, anti-inflammatory, drug potentiator, immune modulator, etc., etc.) and be so useful in medicine (against burns, sprains, wounds and various cardiovascular and circulatory disorders while also increasingly found useful in various "forms" of cancer) that it took on an elixir-like status.

The American medical/pharmaceutical complex simply does not know what to do with multi-use compounds, especially when they are originally derived from natural sources, have so many uses, and are obviously unpatentable. Hence, DMSO has remained very often in a quasi-limbo status as to what it is used for and under what conditions.

It has been approved by the FDA for a specific condition called interstitial cystitis, a type of bladder infection. In practical application, under a Supreme Court ruling, this means that a physician can "legally" use DMSO for any condition he considers to be amenable to treatment with this material.

In terms of cancer, this quite amazing, and essentially non-toxic, compound has been found to play the following roles:

— induction of *apoptosis* (programmed cell death)
— inhibition of metastases *in vitro* and *in vivo*
— induction of cellular differentiation *in vitro*
— increasing of survival rates in human stomach and colon cancer
— direct anti-cancer activity
— enhancement of chemotherapeutic drugs by increased penetration
— scavenging of free radicals/toxic oxygen (e.g., "antioxidant" properties)(22)

Applied topically, orally, or injectably, and being lighter than water, DMSO has the capability of transporting virtually anything with which it is complexed to far reaches of the body, to penetrate tumor "shells," and to cross the "blood/brain barrier." As such, it is known to be of benefit in dealing with cancer metastases in the brain.

DR. BURZYNSKI AND 'ANTINEOPLASTONS' — RESPECT FOR AN UPSTART

Antineoplaston therapy is an excellent example of a naturally derived treatment advanced by a mainstream physician/scientist operating outside the clubby atmosphere of Cancer Inc. The latter does not like to be challenged, economically or conceptually, and will vigorously fight any such interloper.

Only this attitude can explain the enormous efforts mounted by the American medical/governmental establishment to attempt to utterly crush Polish physician/ biochemist Stanislaw Burzynski MD, PhD of Houston TX, a medical pioneer in the finest tradition. (*see Chapter XVIII*).

As we wrote these lines, Dr. Burzynski had scored an impressive victory -- a US district court trial in Houston TX resulted in a mistrial following his indictment on 75 counts involving the use shipment and billing of cancer patients for antineoplaston therapy.

The trial, coming after four Grand Jury probes and various forms of legal harassments over 14 years, was accompanied by the strange reality that while one agency of the federal government (FDA) was actively suppressing antineoplastons, another, the National Cancer Institute (NCI), was actively studying them.

Antineoplastons may not be a magic-bullet cure for cancer, but — as hundreds of "Dr. B's" doctors can attest — this benign therapy has saved many lives and enhanced longevity in numerous cases, including advanced brain cancer.

In his native Poland, Dr. Burzynski began meticulously researching what he believed to be a "parallel immune system" in the form of a group of peptides (chains of amino acids) isolated from human urine. Following a heroic escape from Communist Poland and his immigration into the United States, he transferred his promising work to a research institute and clinic in Houston, and began securing notable successes.

Then the dam broke: the FDA raided his clinic, removed patient records and found the heroic emigre doctor in violation of various federal statutes. The State of Texas weighed in with a satchelful of charges and counts. Medical insurance companies refused to pay for his "experimental" therapies, however promising.

Enraged, his patients went to court and secured some victories both against insurance companies and the State of Texas. But, for more than a decade, pressures for him to close up shop have been unrelenting. Yet, each new crackdown on "Dr. B" simply has brought more publicity and the harassment of this physician/scientist has been a primary stimulus for medical reform in the USA. (*see Chapter XVIII*).

Dr. Burzynski has repeatedly published on, and appeared at international research bodies concerning, his view that various "antineoplastons" can control various "kinds" of cancer. I have found similar compounds to be highly useful weapons against the malignant process.

In parallel research, carried out by less visible scientists, many more of these naturally occurring protein complexes, called peptides or polypeptides, have been found to have immune-enhancing and anti-cancer properties. Some of these peptides are produced by the thymus gland, some by the spleen and liver, and some by the brain, particularly that portion known as the hypothalamus, at the base of the brain.

As we have seen, these substances are essential to a normally functioning immune system, and all of the cancer-fighting cells, such as the Killer T-cells, receive their instructions by way of these chemical messengers. No cellular immune activity can occur without them.

The study of peptides by establishment research led to the discovery of Interferon and Interleukin II, both of which are immune activating peptides, and both of which are currently in use by conventional oncologists (*see Chapter VI*). These substances may be derived from sources other than human urine, particularly the glands of animals. As such, several oral glandular products are available today, such as thymus tablets or capsules, through health food stores and other legitimate outlets.

Oddly enough, Dr. Burzynski's careful scientific work with urine-derived "antineoplastons" in a left-handed kind of way has been among those things which have rekindled interest in one of the most ancient forms of medicine still practiced by people in many lands:

Self-consumption of one's own urine. Before readers gag at the suggestion, it should be noted that some 400 medically useful compounds exist in this watery substance.

Some derivatives of urine are used by mainstream doctors, such as urokinase, a clot-dissolving agent. It may be of interest to the many women taking female hormones that the most widely consumed of these products, Premarin, was first extracted from the urine of pregnant mares (hence the derivation of the name from *Pre*gnant *Mar*e's Ur*ine*) until the pharmaceutical industry, true to form, found a way to synthesize and, of course, patent it. So the idea of finding substances of therapeutic value in urine is not new, nor is it entirely unconventional.

UREA — NATURALLY

The natural substance *urea* is found in abundant quantity in the urine of humans and other mammals, and results from the breakdown of nitrogen-rich foods, mainly proteins. It is used in medicine conventionally as a diuretic, to remove excess fluid from the body, and as an ingredient in many topical medications for the skin. In many alternative care clinics, as well as some conventional care facilities in other lands, it is used in anti-cancer protocols.

The use of urea against cancer is not new, the compound having been used in medicine for over a century. In developing countries, where sophisticated diagnostic equipment, radiation units, and advanced hospital facilities are often not available, simple and inexpensive treatments such as urea can be of great benefit.

For example, in India in 1977, 20 cases of advanced cancer of the cervix were treated with intratumor injections of urea along with topical or surface applications of a urea ointment. All of these were cases which had advanced beyond the point of being helped by surgery. There was a 50-75% reduction in size of growth in seven of these patients (35% of the total patients treated), a 25-50% reduction in tumor size in another seven patients (another 35% of the total), and a conversion from stage III to stage I in three patients (15% of the total), showing a total improvement rate of 85%.

In several of these patients there was a dramatic reduction of the size of metastatic lymph nodes in the pelvis. Other types of cancer successfully treated in this study were osteosarcoma, cancer of the penis, and metastatic cancer of the liver.**(23)**

In Athens, several impressive studies were carried out in the 1970s by E.D. Danopoulos MD, showing nearly 100% effectiveness of urea against various cancers of the eye when it was injected locally into tumors.**(24,25,26)** Dr. Danopoulos also found urea to be effective in liver malignancies, both in primary tumors (hepatomas) and in secondary or metastatic cancers. He found that liver tumors were the only internal cancers which would respond to urea when given by mouth. This was thought to be due to direct absorption from the intestine into the portal (vein to the liver) circulation, bringing a high concentration of urea to the liver.

Other cancers of internal organs, he found, had to be treated by direct infusions of urea into arteries serving those organs. Over half of his liver cancer patients had complete reductions of both liver size and tumors within the liver; many more had partial reductions; and many patients had impressive survival times (up to 10 years), considering the usually ominous prognosis of this stage of cancer.**(27)**

In my facility, urea is used in all cases of malignant involvement of the liver, and it has shown some benefit in most of these.

Once more, we have a product that is abundantly available, non-toxic, completely safe, effective, inexpensive and. of course, unpatentable — and therefore not meeting the criteria of Cancer Inc.

AZELAIC ACID — FEARED BY CANCER INC.

Azelaic acid is a non-toxic substance which appears to have a specific effect on malignant melanoma, the most virulent and vicious of all skin cancers. Much of the experimental work on this material was done by Italian researchers in the late 1970s, who showed that it caused regression or reversal of advancing edges of skin lesions, flattening of nodular (bumpy) areas, and progressive lightening of pigmentation of malignant melanomas.**(28)**

They demonstrated that microscopically there was less malignant activity after treatment with azelaic acid, either topically (applied to the skin) or taken by mouth. Apparently this unusual substance has a specific killing or inhibiting effect on melanoma cells, and this effect is due to its inhibition of tyrosinase, an enzyme unique and vital to melanoma cells, while not adversely affecting normal cells.**(29,30)** These patient studies included some with metastatic cancer and some patients who were considered terminal showed improvement. Research has shown the selective effect as killing or inhibiting the growth of malignant melanoma cells with no effect on normal cells *in vitro*.**(31)**

Other effects of azelaic acid include its interference with the way certain cancer cells acquire their energy, namely anaerobic (without oxygen) glycolysis (breakdown of sugar), which disturbs vital processes in the mitochondria (energy center) of the cancer cell. These cancer-killing effects of azelaic acid are magnified by the addition of 1-carnitine, a recently discovered member of the B-complex family.**(32)**

Early literature on azelaic acid indicated that it was not found in nature except in rancid fats and oils, but some more recent studies have shown that it occurs normally in blood and urine, and is found in the bark of poplar trees.**(33)**

My experience with the use of this fascinating substance has been favorable, and roughly parallels that of the Italian clinic, *Instituto Dermatologico San Gallicano,* Rome, where most of the aforementioned studies took place. However, my experience has been with far fewer patients and those with different stages of the disease. Most of the melanoma patients who have come to me have already been operated on at least once, some several times, and many have already developed metastases.

It is interesting to note that when I first became interested in azelaic acid about 15 years ago — thanks to investigative journalist Wayne Martin — I found that the chemical companies which made it would not sell it to doctors! A chemist, such as a high school chemistry teacher, could readily obtain this material, but a physician could not.

The FDA had issued warnings to chemical companies not to sell azelaic acid — completely non-toxic to humans — to physicians because it was considered a new drug and the effect on humans was considered unknown.

While not admitted by the FDA, patentability again enters the picture. An Italian patent was issued to the director of the clinic in Rome, but it limited the use of azelaic acid to *non-cancerous* conditions. The exact legal status in this country of this harmless substance remains in limbo, but it is obvious that the cancer establishment is not only not interested in it, but as with so many other useful substances, is bent upon preventing its use by patients unfortunate enough to develop malignant melanoma.

Which brings to light another huge obstacle to progress against cancer, and against most of the killer diseases in this country: the unwavering insistence by the US medical establishment, including Cancer Inc., that research in any other country is somehow unreliable. Here we are witnessing the scientific arrogance that only US research is acceptable to the FDA and other arms of the medical-industrial complex. By refusing to accept the results of valid research from other countries, progress in this country, such as it is, proceeds at a snail's pace but with an enormous price tag.

The current total expenses for developing a single drug escalates to well over $200 million by the time the multitude of FDA requirements is met, the cost of which, of course, is ultimately borne by the consumer. And, naturally, drug companies have no interest in any medication or substance which is cheap, natural, non-synthesized, and unpatentable.

Consequently we have, in azelaic acid, just such a product which has, I believe, great potential in the management and control of malignant melanoma, but which remains one of the many natural substances feared and suppressed by Cancer Inc.

BUTYRATE — UNPATENTABLE GODSEND

The butyrates and butyric acid are naturally occurring, non-toxic compounds found in butter and cottage cheese. They have been shown to have inhibiting effects on certain "types" of cancer, namely lymphomas, some leukemias, multiple myeloma, and neuroblastomas. There is a wealth of scientific data in the world literature demonstrating the anti-cancer effects of these substances.

Their first recorded use against cancer, to my knowledge, was in 1933, when Dr. James Watson of Glasgow, Scotland, successfully treated a case of cancer of the cervix with butyric acid. This discovery was made in the course of cleaning up the area of the cervix in preparation for surgery, using capsules containing the butyric acid powder and inserting them into the patient's vagina.(34)

Dr. Watson found that these capsules were effective in clearing up this as well as other malignant growths such as cancers of the stomach, rectum and colon, as well as papillomas. He concluded that butyric acid and its salts were highly selective in their destructive effect on cancer cells and not harmful to normal tissues. Of the various preparations he used, he found the butyrates in powdered form the most effective.

From the late 1960s on, the butyrates were investigated both in laboratory animals and in humans, showing beneficial effects against several "types" of cancer, including multiple myeloma and melanoma.(35,36,37)

Clinical trials using sodium butyrate were carried out in the 1970s in Amsterdam, where patients with advanced metastatic neuroblastomas were treated with this substance. Other studies followed, and it was shown that large doses of this material, up to 10 grams per day, produced no clinically detectable toxicity. This demonstrated a wide margin of safety.(38)

Cecil Pitard MD, an immunologist in Knoxville TN, after having been diagnosed with malignant lymphoma, and after having been told by his fellow physicians that conventional oncology had no more to offer him, decided to research the literature and found an abundance of information about alternative treatments for this disease. Among these were the butyrates, which he incorporated into his treatment program.

Dr. Pitard also used concurrent stimulation of the immune system with injections of staphage lysate, a derivative of the Staphylococcus, along with Indocin, an anti-inflammatory drug, to counteract the toxic effects of the decay and death of tumor masses. He found this combination highly effective in reducing and finally eradicating the many tumor masses in his own body, then going on to successfully treat other patients with lymphoma with this combination, using 10 grams of sodium butyrate daily.

Pitard presented his findings on the use of butyrates at the First Annual Symposium on Man and his Environment in Dallas February 12, 1983, after having been rejected several times by other scientific and medical organizations.

My experience with the Pitard Protocol (or variations of it) against lymphomas is that the butyrates, used together with a total metabolic program, have shown favorable results in most cases.

Another promising area of use of the butyrates is in the acute leukemias. This group of blood cell malignancies is, in my experience, the most unresponsive of all cancers to either conventional or unconventional therapy, with some notable exceptions. So anything that offers even a glimmer of hope to acute leukemia patients (often children) would be a godsend.

After demonstrating the effect of butyrate on leukemia cells in the test tube, Russian scientists treated a five-year-old boy with acute myelogenous leukemia after he had become refractory to standard chemotherapy. They used a continuous intravenous administration of a 2% sodium butyrate solution in 500 ml. of IV solution daily for 10 days. This resulted in remarkable changes in the abnormal white blood cells, called myeloblasts.

These steadily decreased, and 15 days after the initiation of the butyrate, there were no abnormal cells detectable; they had been replaced by normal mature white blood cells. There were no toxic effects noted either during or after the butyrate infusion. The patient was discharged, but returned two weeks later because of the reappearance of myeloblasts. He was then placed on chemotherapy (Vincristine, Cytosine arabinoside, and 6-thioguanine) plus butyrate.

Apparently as a result of the chemotherapy, he had a severe drop in his white blood cell count, followed by sepsis (blood stream infection) and death.(39) While this child unfortunately succumbed (probably to chemotherapy), his case demonstrated some of the remarkable properties of butyrate: to eliminate myeloblasts (immature cells from bone marrow) from the circulating blood in a patient with acute leukemia, to reduce the myeloblasts in the bone marrow from 80% to 20%, to replace myeloblasts with more normal mature myeloid cells, and to do all this without toxicity.

One of the foremost authorities on the butyrates in this country is Professor K. N. Prasad of the University of Colorado, who conducted an extensive review of the literature on the subject. Dr. Prasad found that sodium butyrate had efficacy against neuroblastoma tumors while being essentially non-toxic.(40)

Quoting Dr. Prasad in 1980: "An ideal tumor therapeutic agent must satisfy the following conditions: (a) it should be nontoxic to normal proliferating cells; and (b) it kills and/or differentiates tumor cells in large numbers either directly or by stimulating the host's immune system. At present, most of the currently used tumor therapeutic agents do not possess the above properties of an ideal tumor therapeutic agent. There is no doubt that extensive use of multiple drugs and/or ionizing radiation has produced an increased number of five-year survivors in certain types of human tumors, but the risk of second tumors and other toxic side effects of treatment remains in these survivors. Therefore, the present use of aggressive therapy, involving near lethal doses of immunosuppressive agents, cannot be considered desirable. Recent studies indicate that sodium butyrate possesses both properties of an ideal tumor therapeutic agent."(41)

With this much going for it, one would think that butyrate would find some place in the conventional arsenal of weapons against cancer. But obviously it does not qualify, according to the bizarre standards of modern chemotherapy; i.e., (1) it is a naturally-occurring substance, (2) it is non-toxic, (3) it selectively kills cancer cells without damaging normal cells, (4) it is not patentable, and (5) it is inexpensive.

Research at the American Biologics-Mexico Hospital in Tijuana has demonstrated regression of symptoms and tumors in patients with lymphocytic lymphomas with the oral administration of sodium and potassium butyrate in conjunction with a total metabolic program. The mechanism by which this occurs appears to be the "differentiation" — or return toward normal — of undifferentiated cancer cells by unmasking the genetic material of the cell.

Ongoing research at AB-Mexico against a variety of leukemias and lymphomas has shown encouraging results.**(42)**

My own experience with the butyrates, when used against a variety of cancers, and when used in conjunction with an overall metabolic program, confirms the foregoing observations.

HYDRAZINE SULFATE —
COLD-SHOULDERED BY US ORTHODOXY

Hydrazine sulfate is a common chemical substance used initially as an ingredient in rocket fuel and later developed by Joseph Gold MD, of the Syracuse Cancer Research Institute, as an anti-cancer drug.

It has been in limited clinical use since 1973, designated as an Investigational New Drug by the FDA. Most of the hydrazine research in this country, both in animals and in humans, has been done by Dr. Gold.

He based his work upon Otto Warburg's Nobel Prize-winning discovery that cancer thrives on an abnormal form of metabolism called "anaerobic glycolysis," or the fermentation of sugar in the absence of oxygen. It was theorized that depriving cancer cells of glucose could stop the growth of tumors, and hydrazine has just this capability.

In the early 1970s Dr. Gold found that hydrazine inhibited the growth of cancers in rats, including melanoma, lymphoma and leukemia.**(43,44)**

Clinical results on late stage cancer patients have shown a high degree of positive results from the oral administration of hydrazine sulfate, in terms of subjective response as well as antitumor response. In a study of 84 terminal and pre-terminal cancer patients, 70%, or 59 patients, improved subjectively while 17%, or 14 patients, showed accompanying anti-tumor response.

Subjective responses included increased appetite, weight gain, or stabilization of weight, improvement in strength and performance and decreased pain. Objective responses included reduction of tumor size, disappearance of cancer-related medical complications and more than one year of a stable condition. The side effects if any, were mild. No serious side effects, such as bone marrow suppression, were encountered.**(45)**

These findings were supported by a more extensive Russian study over five years involving 225 terminal cancer patients who had ceased to respond to all other modes of cancer therapy and in whom hydrazine was used as the sole treatment, given at least six weeks following any previous therapy.

In this resistant or refractory group of patients, 65.2% had positive subjective responses and 44% had accompanying anti-tumor responses. Subjective responses included improvement of appetite, weight gain, weight stabilization, disappearance or reduction of severe weakness, improvement in performance status, reduction or complete elimination of pain, and clearing of cancer-related findings and return to normal of laboratory tests.

As with Dr. Gold's study, reduction in size of tumors, and stabilized condition for two months or longer, with some long-term survivals, were noted. Side effects in this study were also mild, consisting of reversible nausea, dry skin, itching and tingling of fingers and toes particularly if treatment was continued for two months without interruption. These symptoms could be relieved or eliminated by reducing the dosage of the hydrazine or temporarily stopping the drug. There were no serious toxic effects, such as suppression of bone marrow or decreased blood cell formation.

Other clinical studies, including some that were "double-blind, placebo-controlled," at Harbor-UCLA Medical Center, consistently demonstrated appetite improvement and weight gain or maintenance of weight in the hydrazine-treated cancer patients, as compared to "controls," or patients receiving the placebo. In one of these studies, all of the cancer patients were far enough advanced to have suffered weight loss, and all had been heavily pre-treated. Hydrazine sulfate appears to be able to interfere with the abnormal sugar metabolism of cancer cells and to reverse the cachexia or wasting associated with advanced cancer.(46,47)

A large Russian study involving over 700 patients with many different "types" of cancer showed significant improvement in weight and/or weight-maintenance, stabilization of disease, and tumor reduction. This study indicated that hydrazine had the best results with Hodgkin's disease, neuroblastoma, cancers of the breast, larynx, and desmosarcoma.(48)

In all of these studies, hydrazine sulfate has been shown to accomplish something that no other drug or conventional treatment modality has been able to do — namely, to reverse cachexia, along with its accompanying loss of appetite, weight loss and profound weakness. Add to these a significant degree of tumor reduction, stabilization of disease, with lack of toxicity, and one would think the cancer establishment would be clamoring for this substance.

Instead, the National Cancer Institute has, for many years, constantly belittled and disparaged hydrazine, and discouraged its use in cancer patients. Again we seem to be witnessing a pattern of irrational behavior on the part of the establishment similar to that observed with other useful substances. And again, the only reasons I can come up with are that hydrazine is, like all the others: (1) readily available, (2) inexpensive, (3) non-toxic, (4) effective, and (5) unpatentable.

My experience in practice with hydrazine sulfate has been more or less comparable to that of most of the clinical studies in the literature: that is, in cancer patients who have trouble with appetite, weight loss, weakness, muscle wasting and other signs of cachexia, there has been fairly consistent improvement.

CELLULAR THERAPY — LESS BIZARRE TODAY

Some "natural" anti-cancer protocols — implemented where such is legal — may include what is generally called "live cell" or "cellular" therapy, known in Europe for more than 70 years but just now beginning to be heard about in the USA.

This treatment is the subcutaneous or intramuscular injection of salt suspensions of living cellular material from birth-related tissues (embryonic, fetal, placental) from animals.

While originally advanced early in this century as a kind of natural hormonal treatment either for problems of fertility/sterility and for the management of chronic skin conditions, live cell therapy swiftly took on the reputation of being a longevity method for the rich and famous. While it is true that many of the latter, seeking everlasting health and better sex lives, trekked to the late Paul Niehans' Clinique La Prairie in Switzerland, a major world center of this kind of medicine, cellular therapy has far greater ramifications.

Modern-day exponents find that birth-related endocrine tissue apparently has a "balancing" effect on the whole range of hormones in the body as well as a manifest capability of restoring or improving damaged organs and tissues across species lines. Inasmuch as the endocrine or hormonal system impacts on every other system of the body, and inasmuch as hormonal imbalance is a frequent factor in cancer in particular and chronic disease in general, there is at least a sound biochemical rationale for its use.**(49,50)**

US orthodox research — which has deftly changed the name of these treatments to "fetal-cell transplantation therapy" and similar designations — has primarily focused on Parkinson's, muscular dystrophy and some rare inherited disorders, which indeed have responded dramatically to such treatments.

Cellular therapy proponents find live cells to be of benefit in cancer in two ways:

First, fibroblasts from umbilical cords seem to induce production of messenger-cell interleukins, which may have a direct effect on cancer.

Second, organs and tissues damaged by the cancer process or by its orthodox therapy may be healed, enhanced or repaired through embryonic matching tissues.**(51)**

Most foreign clinics are using birth-related tissues from bovine sources, though some prefer shark. It is evident that such tissues from the mammalian/viviparous species are useful.

Adjunctive to live cell therapy frequently is the intramuscular administration of glandular extracts or even oral consumption of powdered glandulars.

Lyophilized or freeze-dried injectable cellular suspensions are also commercially available from Europe though cellular therapy purists argue that the same, while often useful, are really "dead" cells.

As it is, live cell therapy is another treatment approach in limbo in the USA, at least outside the rigid confines of a few research universities utilizing tissue from aborted human fetuses — it is not a drug in the real meaning of the word, but is rather a technique. The raw material is massively abundant in the world today and there can be no meaningful patent on its use. It remains, hence, "unproven" — which is to say, mostly inaccessible to the general public.

REFERENCES

1. Asai, Kazuhiko, *Organic Gemanium, a Medical Godsend.* Tokyo: Kogaskusha, 1977.

2. Kumano, Nobuko, *et al., Sci. Rep. Res. Inst., Tohuku Univ.* 25, 1978.

3. Kidd, P., "Germanium-132: homeostatic normalizer and immunostimulant: a review of its preventive and therapeutic efficacy." *Intl. Clin. Nutr. Rev.* 7 (1), 1987.

4. Aso, H., *et al.,* "Introduction of interferon and activation of NK cells and macrophages in mice by oral administration of GE-132, an organic germanium compound." *J. Microbiol. and Immunol.* 29, 1985.

5. "She 'turned political' and beat three-week prognosis by 4 years!" *The Choice,* XVII:2, 1991.

6. Littarru, G.P., *et al.,* in K. Folkers and Y. Yamamura, *eds., Biomedical and Clinical Aspects of Coenzyme Q,* Vol. 4. Amsterdam: Elsevier Science, 1984.

7. Folkers, Karl, *et al., Research Communications in Chemical Pathology and Pharmacology* 19:3, 1978.

8. Lockwood, Knud, *et al.,* "Partial and complete remission of breast cancer in patients in relation to dosage of Coenzyme Q10." *Biochem. and Biophys. Res. Comm.* 199:3, 1994.

9. Keller, H., "Carnivora: immunomodulator and cytostatic. Study of treatment of Carnivora in patients with advanced malignant disease." Nordhalben, Germany: *Carnivora Forschungs Gmbh,* 1994.

10. Walker, Morton, "The Carnivora cure for cancer, AIDS and other pathologies." *Townsend Letter for Doctors,* Part I. June, 1991; Part II, May, 1992.

11. Walker, Morton, "Profile of Helmut Keller MD, the physician who reverses colitis and chronic and infective degenerative diseases." *Raum & Zeit,* June, 1991.

12. Walker, Morton, "The Carnivora . . ." Part II, *op. cit.*

13. Kreher, B., *et al.,* "Structure elucidation of plumbagin analogues from *Dionaea muscipula* and their immunomodulating activities in vitro and in vivo." International Symposium: Molecular Recognition, Sopron, Hungary, Aug. 24-27, 1988.

14. Walker, Morton, "The Carnivora . . . " Part II, *op. cit.*

15. Lane, I.W. and Comac, L., *Sharks Don't Get Cancer.* Garden City Park NY: Avery, 1992.

16. Lane, W., and Miller, M., "A comparison of shark cartilage and bovine cartilage." *Townsend Letter for Doctors & Patients,* April 1996.

17. Prudden, J.F., "Position paper on cartilage therapy and comparison of bovine and shark cartilage; most commonly asked questions and other areas of comparison." *Townsend Letter for Doctors & Patients,* April 1996.

18. Lerner, M., and Flint, D., *Does Cartilage Cure Cancer? The Shark and Bovine Cartilage Controversy: an Independent Assessment.* Bolinas, CA: Commonweal, 1995.

19. Kirchhof, D., and Kirchhof, E., *The Successful Use of Bovine Tracheal Cartilage in the Treatment of Cancer.* Belgrade MT: Kriegel and Associates, 1995.

20. "A shark cartilage IND." *The Choice*, XXI:2, 1995.

21. Halstead, B.W., and Youngberg, S.A., *The DMSO Handbook.* Colton, CA: Golden Quill, 1981.

22. Boik, J., *Cancer and Natural Medicine.* Princeton, MN: Oregon Medical Press, 1995.

23. Gandhi, G.M., *et al.,* "Urea in the management of advanced malignancies." *J. Surg. Oncol.* 9, 139-146, 1977.

24. Danopoulos, E.D., *et al.,* "Urea in the treatment of epibulbar malignancies." *Br. J. Ophthalmol.* 59: 282-7, 1975.

25. Danopoulos, E.D., and Danopoulos, I.E., "Effects of urea treatment in combination with curettage in extensive periophthalmic malignancies." *Ophthalmologica* 179: 52-61, 1979.

26. Danopoulos, E.D., *et. al.,* "Effects of urea treatment in malignancies of the conjunctiva and cornea." *Ophthalmologica* 178: 198-203, 1979.

27. Danopoulos, E.D., "Eleven years' experience of oral urea treatment in liver malignancies." *Clin. Oncol.* 7: 281-9, 1981.

28. Nazarro-Porro, M., *et al., Lancet,* 1 (8178) 1109-11, May 24, 1980.

29. Nazarro-Porro, M., and Passi, S., "Identification of tyrosinase inhibitors in cultures of pityrosporum." *J. Invest. Dermatol.* 71: 205-08, 1978.

30. Nazarro-Porro, M., *et al.,* "Effect of dicarboxylic acids on lentigo maligne." *J. Invest. Dermatol.* 72: 296-305, 1979.

31. Geier, G., *et al.,* "Effect of azelaic acid on the growth of melanoma cell cultures." *Hautarzt.* 37: 146-8, 1986.

32. Ward, B.J., *et al.,* "Effect of 1-carnitine on cultured murine melanoma cells exposed to azelaic acid." *J. Invest. Dermatol.* 86: 438-41, 1986.

33. Neesby, T. Personal communication, ref. *Pochvovedennie* 44-51, 1980.

34. Watson, J., "Butyric acid in the treatment of cancer." *Lancet*, 746-8, April, 1933.

35. Anger, G., *et al.,* "Treatment of multiple myeloma with a new cytostatic agent — butyric acid." *Deutsch Med. Wochenschr.* 94: 2495-500, 1969.

36. Nordenberg, J., *et al.,* "Growth inhibition of murine melanoma by butyric acid and DMSO." *Exp. Cell Res.* 162: 77-85, 1986.

37. Nordenberg, J., *et al.,* "Biochemical and ultrastructural alterations accompany the anti-proliferative effect of butyrate on melanoma cells." *Br. J. Cancer.* 55: 493-7, 1987.

38. Prasad, K., "Butyric acid: a small fatty acid with diverse biological functions." *Life Sciences* 27: 1351-8, 1980.

39. Novogrodsky, A., *et al.,* "Effect of polar organic compounds on leukemic cells. Butyrate-induced partial remission of acute myelogenous leukemia in a child." *Cancer* 51: 9-14, 1983.

40. Prasad, K., and Sinka, P., "Effect of sodium butyrate on mammalian cells in culture: a review." *In Vitro* 12: 125-32, 1976.

41. Prasad, K., 1980, *op. cit.*

42. Bradford, R., *et al.,* monograph. *Butyric Acid Therapy as a New Adjunctive in the Treatment of Degenerative Diseases.* Chula Vista CA: Bradford Research Institute, 1986.

43. Gold, J., "Inhibition of W256 IM carcinoma in rats by administration of hydrazine sulfate" *Oncol.* 25: 66-71, 1971.

44. Gold, J., "Inhibition by hydrazine sulfate, etc., of growth of W256 IM carcinoma, melanoma, lymphosarcoma, and solid leukemia." *Oncol.* 27: 69-80, 1973.

45. Gold, J., "Use of hydrazine sulfate in terminal and pre-terminal cancer patients; results of IND study in 84 evaluable patients." *Oncol.* 32: 1-10, 1975.

46. Chlebowski, R., *et al.,* "Influence of hydrazine sulfate on abnormal carbohydrate metabolism in cancer patients with weight loss." *Cancer Res.* 44: 857-61, 1984.

47. Chlebowski, R., *et al.,* "Influence of hydrazine sulfate on abnormal carbohydrate metabolism in cancer patients with weight loss; a placebo-controlled clinical experience." *Cancer* 59: 406-10, 1987.

48. Filov, V., *et al.,* "Results of clinical evaluation of hydrazine sulfate." *Vopr. Onkol.* 36: 7821-726, 1990.

49. Kuhnau, W.W., *Live-Cell Therapy: My Life with a Medical Breakthrough.* Tijuana, Mexico: Artes Graficas de Baja California, 1983, 1992.

50. Schmid, Franz, *Cell Therapy, a New Dimension of Medicine.* Switzerland: Ott, 1993.

51. Culbert, M.L., *Live Cell Therapy for the 21st Century.* Chula Vista CA: The Bradford Foundation, 1993.

Chapter XIV
THE BALANCING OF ENERGY —
Homeopathy, Energetics, Wellness and Illness

In 1994, yet another case for the two-century-old practice of homeopathy became so apparent that even a standard medical journal, *The Lancet,* observed (through California pediatrician Carol D. Berkowitz):

> *"Despite . . . barriers to universal acceptance of homeopathy, physicians should maintain an open mind about potential benefits. Although we have often relied on drugs such as antibiotics to manage disorders such as diarrhea, the emergence of resistant organisms may necessitate a change in strategies."*(1)

She was responding to a *Lancet* article in which homeopathic dilutions had successfully managed acute diarrhea in Nicaraguan children.(2) Such research — based on the Western "scientific" model of medicine — had come on the heels of credible information in standard journals which described homeopathic victories over allergies and hay fever(3) and an earlier 12-scientist, four-country study in which a homeopathic dilution so tiny not a molecule was microscopically recoverable had apparently stimulated an immune response in white blood cells.(4)

All such research has pointed to the rapid resurgence of homeopathy, a medical discipline developed in the 18th century by a German, Samuel Hahnemann, which at one point became *the* major form of medicine practiced in the USA (fighting a life-and-death struggle with standard medicine, or allopathy(5) and which has been alive and kicking in various parts of the world for generations.

Homeopathy became an odd-man-out in American medicine almost entirely because it posed a severe economic challenge to drug-based allopathic medicine:

Under homeopathic theory and practice, minuscule dilutions of medicines or tinctures, from plant, mineral or animal origin, which would cause pathological symptoms in a healthy person if given in larger amounts, are provided ill people at tiny levels against the same symptoms. This is a restatement of the ancient medical view of Hippocrates and Paracelsus that "like cures like," later described by Hahnemann as "the law of similars." If such symptoms are so treated, goes the theory, then the disturbance in the "vital force" which caused the disease symptoms in the first place will be corrected and recovery results.

Modern-day proponents of Eastern philosophical and medical techniques will instantly perceive that what Hahnemann was talking about in 18th-century Europe was simply a Westernized version of ancient Asian thought made more palatable for the Western mind.

For the resurgence of homeopathy — including the utilizing, now, of hundreds of homeopathic remedies against numerous symptoms, including those of cancer — has been paralleled by the advance into Western medical thinking of Asian healing techniques.

Whether described as "pranic healing" (from the Indian *prana*) or various Chinese techniques utilizing *chi* (or *qi*) or the Japanese *reiki* (boundless vital energy), or, in Western parlance, homeopathy, all such approaches boil down to a central concept:

All health and disease — indeed, at the philosophical level, all reality — results from the balance or imbalance of pure energy (Hahnemann's "vital force") so that either wellness or illness results.

While Western allopathic medicine came to hate homeopathy with a vengeance it could hardly deny the reality that virtually all Western medicine conceptually dates back to Hippocrates (who taught the holism of man and nature and believed in a vital curative force) and to a lesser but real extent Paracelsus, who also stressed a vital force.

This is not to say that homeopathy "cures" cancer. However, I am aware of one anecdotal case after another in which homeopathic dilutions at the very least reduced or ameliorated various symptoms of cancer which is, after all, a systemic or total-body malignant process of many manifestations.

Homeopathic preparations have also been useful in ridding the body of toxins and residuals from previous diseases which are obstacles to healing.

While my practice is not primarily homeopathy, I do use some homeopathic remedies as permitted by my homeopathic license. Some of my patients are already taking homeopathic remedies when they come to my facility, and I certainly do not discourage their continued use, there being thousands of these remedies from 200 years of homeopathic research, including an official US Homeopathic Pharmacopoeia, to choose from.

A major reason for my support of the practice of homeopathy is that these preparations cannot possibly do harm. There is no way that the minuscule dilutions of substances used in homeopathy can cause any damage to patients. One of the principles advanced by Hippocrates, and later by Sir William Osler, a giant of early Western medicine, was "above all, do no harm."

Modern drug-oriented medicine seems to have forgotten this basic principle of practice, with literally thousands dying annually from the use or misuse of drugs, including and especially the toxic chemotherapeutic drugs.

It is a curious phenomenon that the medical "quackbusters," who support the drug industry, have little to say about homeopathy other than insisting that its premises don't hold up.

Yet some of our modern medical methodologies are clearly based upon the principles of homeopathy. The present-day treatment of allergies with minute doses of the offending substance and the use of vaccines (diluted preparations of killed bacteria, attenuated viruses or other disease-causing organisms) against infections, through the production of antibodies, are clear reflections of homeopathy's "law of similars."

Today's homeopathy — backed by satellite communication between homeopathic doctors, who are trained to study both physical and mental symptoms to design an overall profile of a patient, and to seek out the most effective dilutions of the most effective, usually oral, tinctures — cannot be separated from the appearance in the West of "energy" or "energetic" medicine.

The Eastern approach, on the other hand, utilizes such techniques as exercise and relaxation, meditation, touch, acupuncture, massage, the laying on of hands and faith healing. Some of these, in turn, inevitably carry us into the area of the mind and attitudes (*see Chapter XV*) — that is to say, the mind/spirit elements of the Holistic Triad of mind, spirit and body.

The Western world, notably more materialistic than the Eastern one, has long expressed more interest in the physical effects of a vital force and how it may be quantified and utilized on the physical plane.

For Hahnemann, physical elements — the tiny dilutions of liquids "succussed" or vibrated and diluted to the point that often only their "vital force" remained — could cure disease, and that was enough. There was no need to fit this visible reality into a religious or philosophical system. So homeopathy surged ahead in the Western world as a physical form of medicine despite the lack of any well-understood explanation of exactly how it "worked."

Just as homeopathy was at its zenith in the Western world, other Western trends were looking at related areas of "energy" or "energetic" medicine, usually built on the ideas of bioelectricity, electromagnetism, biomagnetism, and magnetic energy.

The development of mechanical means to balance or influence electromagnetic energy (held by some to be *the* vital force of the universe) led both to new diagnostics and ahead-of-their-time microscopes (the controversial devices of Royal Rife in the United States are among the better known) and any number of machines said to be capable of changing frequencies in that force.

Wilhelm Reich's theory of *orgone energy* and *bions* eventually gave way to the mind-body therapy now called *bioenergetics*. In France, Antoine Priore's "Priore ray" allegedly altered magnetic fields to "cure" cancer but was suppressed by French authorities, as was the case with "Rifeian" technology in the USA.(6)

The use of industrial magnets against disease, including cancer, has been advanced by several experts, some with credible results,(7) and a California research institute developed a way to change cancer cell polarity through "accelerated charges."(8)

From serious quarters there is now information which describes the human body itself as a "closed electrical circuit," an energy-producing field itself within a greater field of energy (planet Earth) within a greater energy field (the cosmos).(9,10) These are latter-day statements by Western thinkers in a Western "scientific" mold of ancient Eastern concepts.

The field is, of course, wide open to chicanery and quackery, but — abuses aside — many research roads are now leading, through Western science, to a validation of eastern philosophical concepts.

Inasmuch as physics is a scientific discipline which increasingly relies nearly as much on the unknown as on the known, with both the demonstration and theorization of not only sub-atomic but possibly even sub-sub-atomic particles — the concept of a universal "vital force" or underlying energy field as the wellspring of all existence is far more credible today, even to the Western-trained scientist, than was the case a few decades ago.

And, as Dr. Berkowitz said in *The Lancet,* given the threat of antibiotic-resistant infections — quite aside from the growing presence of the chronic killer diseases of civilization — it is up to physicians to "maintain an open mind about potential benefits."

This is why I generally do not oppose the participation of some of my patients in various meditative techniques or other holistic practices as long as it is clear that no such technique or practice is physically endangering their health.

After all, since the days of Hippocrates medicine has been concentrated on two fundamental objectives — saving lives and reducing suffering.

If it is clearly demonstrable that a tiny dilution of *Belladonna,* or an appropriate odor, or a proper frequency from a bioelectric machine of some kind, or a muscular adjustment — or a prayer — can assist in either one of these objectives, then it is "good medicine" to use them.

REFERENCES

1. Berkowitz, C.D., "Homeopathy: keeping an open mind." *Lancet,* Sept. 10, 1994.

2. Jacobs, J., *et al.,* "Treatment of acute childhood diarrhea with homeopathic medicine: a randomized clinical trial in Nicaragua." *Pediatrics* 93, 1994.

3. "Homeopathy: much ado about nothing?" *Consumer Reports,* March 1994.

4. Culbert, M.L., *Medical Armageddon.* San Diego, CA: C&C Communications, 1995.

5. Coulter, H.L., *Divided Legacy: the Conflict between Homeopathy and the American Medical Association.* Richmond, CA: North Atlantic Books, 1973.

6. Culbert, *op. cit.*

7. Philpott, W.H., *Cancer: the Magnetic/Oxygen Answer.* Choctaw, OK: 1994.

8. Bradford, R.W., *et al.,* "The effect of magnetic poles on accelerated charge neutralization of malignant tumors in vivo." Intl. Symp. on Biomagnet., Salve Regina College, Newport RI, June 1, 1989. (Bradford Research Institute)

9. Beasley, V., *Your Electro-Vibratory Body.* Boulder Creek, CO: University of the Trees Press, 1978.

10. Becker, R.O., and Seldon, G., *The Body Electric: Electro-Magnetism and the Foundation of Life.* New York: Morrow, 1986.

Chapter XV
HARNESSING THE MIND
Attitudes, Illness and Wellness

Orthodox medicine likes to call them cases of "spontaneous remissions."

The more religious are happy to call them clear evidence of "faith healing."

I prefer to call them "cases of successful positive thinking," with faith playing a key role in this process.

What we are describing here are those scientifically incredible cases in which advanced cancer patients, beating all the odds — at least the physical ones — and not necessarily doing any better on nutritional therapy than they had on orthodoxy, rally and overcome their disease. Some of them go on to live for decades, essentially cancer-free.

Every doctor has seen such patients, and even assumes some of them will fall into this mysterious category.

There is a higher rate of "spontaneous remissions" in cancer than in any other disease, probably because this multifactorial condition represents a pathology in which mental or emotional factors have such an unusually strong presence.

A huge recent global survey of "spontaneous remissions" (3,500 reports from 800 "standard" medical journals appearing in 20 languages) found that 74 percent of the unexpected-recovery cases were of cancer.[1]

To those of us with a holistic frame of mind we are looking at the three portions of what Eastern philosophical and religious systems call the true healing triad — body, mind and spirit.

The healing of old, let it never be forgotten, was based as much on prayer and ritual — that is, faith and mental imagery — as anything done physically by the physician/priest or shaman. "Laying on of hands," in fact, as depicted in cave paintings, is the earliest description of healing by anyone anywhere.[2]

Until this century, when medicine was prostituted into a "science," and captivated by what some call the Cartesian-Newtonian postulates of the 17th century, which set the standard for the "scientific method," it was clear that a lot of "unscientific" things came into play in the doctor-patient relationship and in the healing process:

The faith of the patient in the doctor, the expressed confidence of the doctor in what he was doing, and the understated determination of both to cooperate together in finding the "cure." This often used to mean the taking of extensive notes by the physician, the jotting down of symptoms, the interest in the practitioner of all aspects of what a patient was feeling, eating and thinking.

With the advent of "scientific" allopathic medicine as the dominant paradigm in this century in the Western world, all such "unmeasurable" elements were usually sidelined, along with such "unquantifiable" approaches as homeopathy, so that "science" could fit medicine into a seemingly "correct" mold.

But, as we approach the end of this millenium, a revolution is occurring which is bringing back into focus the extreme importance of the mind, of faith, of attitudes in the causation, management and control of illness and wellness.

Until recently, official scientific thought over most of this century has regarded mind, body and emotions as separate and distinct entities.

Some students of science and medicine for decades have cast about trying to make the mind-body connection and to present it in a comprehensible way acceptable to the scientific agnostics of this century.

Pioneers along the way were Lawrence LeShan, who detailed emotional and attitudinal connections to cancer, and Carl Simonton, who brought the concept of "guided imagery" into the domestic lexicon.(3,4) But it remained for the biochemically minded to put a full dress on an indescribable concept and come up with a new name.

Enunciated in 1988, this concept turned out to be *psychoneuroimmunology* (PNI), whose somewhat cumbersome term suggests "mind-nerves-immunity," a description of a dynamic process which involves thoughts, attitudes, and their communication with the immune and nervous systems by means of the body's hormones.(5,6)

Some of these hormones — or hormone-like substances — are the neuropeptides, or neurotransmitters, which allow the brain to communicate with virtually every cell in the body. It was once thought that these transmitters were produced only by the central nervous system, but we now know that they are produced by every cell involved in the immune process — more evidence of a highly integrated, highly intelligent system.

We are now also aware of how profoundly our immune systems are altered by emotional and spiritual factors.

PNI — and, now, PNE (*psychoneuroendocrinology*) — are literally out of the medical and biological closet. They help define a discipline in Western semantics which incorporates thought — and faith.

At a 1996 conference, Dr. Herbert Benson, a Harvard Medical School professor and founder of the Mind/Body Medical Institute at Boston's Deaconess Hospital, announced that his years of delving into the area had convinced him that the mind could work "like a drug," particularly when people had a strong faith in God or a higher power.

In a study of numerous patients, clinicians reported that repeating prayers had been seen to lower the heart rate, breathing rate and brain wave activity and in some cases had helped the patients avoid surgery.

Dr. Benson told the conferees:

"Scientific studies demonstrate that, by repeating prayers, words or sounds and passively disregarding other thoughts, many people are able to trigger a specific set of physiological changes . . . Eighty percent of the patients, when given the choice of a word, sound or prayer to repeat, chose prayer. I discovered I was teaching prayer."(7)

A few years before, Larry Dossey MD had reached his own defining moment in assessing the results of a 10-month randomized, "blinded" trial of 393 patients at the University of California-San Francisco Medical School's coronary care unit.

When patients were divided into two groups — one prayed-for *without their knowledge* by members of various faiths and the other left un-prayed-for — it was found that the former group had a significantly reduced "severity score;" that is, it needed far less ventilatory assistance, fewer diuretics and fewer antibiotics.

Dr. Dossey, reviewing the data, recorded how he began to pray for patients — and found that such an activity "worked," though it was not necessarily covered by Blue Cross. Prophetically, he analyzed:

"I reached the conclusion that withholding prayer was the equivalent of withholding any other valid medical treatment."(8)

He went on to discover that at least 130 solidly supported studies existed in English-language medical literature attesting to the ability of prayer to heal.(9)

To the faithful, no explanations are necessary. That God works wonders is not a new discovery to those who believe in the power of prayer.

Such research only confirms a much greater reality: the role of attitudes and faith in health and disease.

The so-called "placebo effect," noted by science for generations, has to do entirely with the non-physical or attitudinal. When a mother takes her trembling child into an unfamiliar dark room and tells him, "You're not afraid; you're a big boy now," she is causing a series of physiological changes within her offspring which, among others, will strengthen his own capacity to convert starch into sugar (the so-called "fight or flight" mechanism.) Simply *believing* he is a "big boy now" — an *attitude* — causes him to take on part of the physical attributes of actually *being* one.

Far more elaborate work has gone on demonstrating the mind-body link.

No small part of it has been advanced by Cleve Backster, a former Navy officer who became a major developer of polygraph techniques and spent 25 years monitoring plants and cellular responses through his Backster Research Foundation.

Researcher Robert B. Stone PhD, closely following Backster's work, wrote *The Secret Life of Your Cells* and Peter Tomkins and Christopher Bird authored *The Secret Life of Plants*. These volumes described in detail some strange findings by Backster.

In a newsletter, Dr. Stone, describing Backster as "the father of primary cell perception," wrote:

> *"The Backster research results must make some scientists lie awake at night. Plants that he monitors with polygraph elements react to such events as shrimp dying in boiling water, germs dying as they hit a urinal's antiseptic, or a person entering the laboratory who is destructive with plants.*
>
> *"The cells that he monitors, usually scraped from a human mouth, react to that person's emotions and actions even when miles away."(10)*

This is another demonstration of what other "mind-body" researchers have begun to call "human intention factor," or HIF, which, medically runs like this:

A doctor's clear intention to help a patient, rather than simply to see the patient at 2 pm and write a prescription, will enhance the healing of the patient. The *intention* of a doctor to engage in healing — and even the colors of the wallpaper in his office — reflect a healing attitude and help assist in it.

While some ramifications of the field lend themselves to ridicule and deceit, the area itself is leading to bright new vistas involving the awesome power of thought.

All of which doubles the responsibility of the physician to add positive thinking to the protocol.

I have seen case after case of the devastating effects of a patient's having been told by a doctor somewhere that "you're terminal, there's nothing more that I can do, and you should go home and get your affairs in order." Such a series of negative statements constitutes a major enhancement of illness and, I firmly believe, has no business in the doctor's office, or mind.

This is not to say that the practitioner need lie to the patient or sugar-coat the seriousness of a disease condition: it *is* a statement that to a logical, feasible and moral extent, everything should be done to strengthen the patient's resolve for victory over disease.

In the modern era, such forward-looking thinkers as Bernie Siegel MD(11) have noted how "difficult" patients — that is, those who do not sit by passively waiting for "doctor" to minister to them, but who aggressively try to take charge of their own healing and irritate the daylights out of doctor and nurse with a seemingly endless flow of questions — are more apt to survive than are their more docile counterparts.

My own experience has been that those patients who, from Day One of a diagnosis, decided to live day-by-day and marshal an inner strength to overcome their life-threatening condition, and who simply refused somebody's prognosis of "six months to live," more often than not had the last laugh.

For no mortal on this planet, however much equipped with the finest scientific gadgetry, truly knows when anyone else is going to die, or under what circumstances. Doctors who coldly pronounce their patients dead within a specific timeframe may often think they simply are being honest — but they are short-changing the patient and increasing illness by instilling desperation.

Furthermore, by pronouncing this "death sentence" these physicians are — perhaps unwittingly — programming their patients to die on a certain date. It has been my experience that when this dire prediction is accepted by the patient (and how many are willing to question the doctor's knowledge and authority?), more often than not, that patient will die on schedule. This, of course, makes the physician look brilliant almost to the point of infallibility.

But I truly believe this phenomenon to be much more a product of the programmable mind than the brilliance of the doctors.

That is why, more and more, we are learning to listen to our patients and to encourage their positive thoughts in every rational, responsible way and not to accept negative and discouraging input *from any source.*

THE CANCER PERSONALITY

Going back in history to the second century AD, Galen, a Greek physician famous for his astute observations, noted that women who tended to be melancholic or pensive had a greater tendency to develop breast cancer.

In dealing with thousands of cancer patients over the years, it has been my observation also that there are certain underlying personality traits which appear to be consistently present in these individuals.

They are typically highly conscientious, caring, hard working, and usually of better than average intelligence. They tend to take on other peoples' burdens and accept extra obligations to such an extent that they leave themselves little time for relaxation or their own pleasurable pursuits. They tend to be "people-pleasers" and apparently have a deep-seated need to make others happy, a commendable personality feature under other circumstances but possibly fatal in this setting.

Typical of the cancer-susceptible personality, or what we now often refer to as the "Type C" personality, is the long-standing suppression of emotions, particularly anger. Usually starting at an early age, these people have held in their hostility and other unacceptable emotions. Most often this feature of one's personality goes back to feelings of rejection by one or both parents. Whether these feelings are justified or not, the result is a lack of closeness with the "rejecting" parent or parents, followed later in life by a similar lack of closeness with spouses and others with whom close relationships would normally develop.

Some of these feelings of rejection are normal and occur at times in all of us at one time or another, but when they become a dominant feature or are chronically present, the risk factors go up. Those at higher risk for cancer tend to develop a sense of loneliness resulting from their having been deprived of affection and acceptance earlier in life, even if this is merely their own perception. These people have a tremendous need for approval and acceptance, developing a high sensitivity to the needs of others while suppressing their own emotional needs.

They become the "caretakers" of the world, showing great compassion for others and going out of their way to care for the needs of others. They are very reluctant to accept care from others, fearing that it might jeopardize their role as caretakers, or fearing that they may appear to have too much self-concern. Throughout their childhood they have typically been taught not to be "selfish" and have taken this to heart.

The cancer-susceptible individual typically bears his/her burdens in silence and without complaint. Burdens of their own, as well as the burdens of others, weigh heavily, often subconsciously, upon these individuals because they — through a lifetime of suppression — internalize their cares, problems and conflicts.

The carefree extrovert, on the other hand, seems to be invulnerable — or at least far less vulnerable to cancer than the caring introvert just described.

STRESS MANAGEMENT

How one reacts to stress is a major factor in the development of most illness, particularly in the area of the so-called "degenerative diseases" — cancer, of course, being included in this category.

Nearly all of the cancer patients I have attended have experienced a highly stressful event — or series of events — usually about two years prior to the establishment of the diagnosis. This traumatic event is often beyond the patient's control, such as the loss of a loved one, loss of a business, job, home, or other major financial disaster.

Major stress, as we have seen, causes suppression of the immune system, and does so more overwhelmingly in the cancer-susceptible personality described above. Thus personal tragedies and excessive levels of stress combine with underlying personality traits to bring on the immune deficiency which allows the cancer to thrive.

For some reason, the cancer victim has lost his/her ability — or sometimes even desire — to cope with the seemingly overwhelming stress burden that has befallen him/her. Often an unresolved conflict dating back to childhood will — if allowed to remain unexpressed and unresolved — manifest itself later in life as a malignant process.

Negative attitudes — sometimes referred to as "toxic emotions" — such as guilt, resentment, animosity, bitterness, and pessimism, must be purged from the patient victimized by these destructive feelings, and replaced with the positives of love, forgiveness and optimism.(12) While doing good for others is always a commendable pursuit, it must not be carried to the extreme or to the point of compulsiveness, and must not take the place of enlightened self-interest, especially in the case of the cancer patient.

One consistent observation in my many years of practice has been that the successful patients have been those who:

1. take charge of their own health rather than being involved in disease management, eliminating the control others seek to impose on them in many areas in addition to that of health.
2. have faith in God or a higher power.
3. are willing to make major changes in their lifestyle, including dietary habits, exposure to chemicals, and work environment.
4. are committed to making changes in their attitudes and behavior, eliminating "toxic emotions" and replacing them with positive ones.
5. have enthusiasm and faith in what they are doing to overcome their disease, whether it be under our recommendations or another similar health-oriented program.
6. can relieve themselves of excessive obligations and responsibilities.
7. are able to talk about their deep-seated problems, conflicts and burdens.

Patients are counseled and encouraged to reclaim their power of healing by first *identifying* the problem, then *addressing* it in a straightforward way, and finally by *dealing* with it openly and honestly. It is always the patient's *response* to his/her particular stress that must be changed more than the stressful situation itself.

All of us, of course, are exposed to stresses, particularly in our Western culture where stress is a way of life. But so often many of us try to change the person or situation causing us the stress and distress, rather than modifying our responses to these factors. True, sometimes situations can be changed — but trying to change people? Good luck.

If visits with one's mother-in-law bring on any of these negative feelings, perhaps it is time to make fewer visits, discontinue them altogether, or distance oneself emotionally from the offending individual.

An excellent book on this subject has recently been written by one of my successful cancer patients, Melanie Zucker.(13) In this book, Melanie describes her battles with the "Power Robbers" in a very readable and motivating manner, culminating in her triumph over all psychological and physical obstacles. I highly recommend this work to anyone struggling with cancer, whether they be following conventional or alternative courses.

To the scientifically oriented, the foregoing comments regarding causation of cancer may seem trifling and immaterial, considering the mountains of scientific data allegedly demonstrating about 1001 causes of this disease. But before dismissing these seemingly off-beat and wild postulations of a medical heretic, consider this: despite the billions expended on finding a cause and cure for cancer over the last half century, the cancer establishment is basically not much closer to solving the puzzle than it was 40 to 50 years ago.

So why not give at least some consideration to "non-establishment" points of view? Put more succinctly, since no other theories have worked, why not try ours?

The brightest moment in therapy for a "terminal" patient, after all, occurs when, following extensive examination by stunned diagnosticians, he is told that he has seemed to have undergone a "spontaneous remission."

REFERENCES

1. Regan, B., and Hershberg, C., *Spontaneous Remission: An Annotated Biography.* Sausalito, CA: Institute of Noetic Sciences, 1993.
2. Culbert, M.L., *Medical Armageddon.* San Diego, CA: C & C Communications, 1995.
3. LeShan, L., *You Can Fight for Your Life: Emotional Factors in the Causation of Cancer.* New York: Evans, 1977.
4. Simonton, C., *et al., Getting Well Again.* New York: Bantam, 1986.

5. Solomon, G.E., *Psychoneuroimmunology.* New York: Academic Press, 1987.

6. Rogers, M.P., *et al.,* "The influence of the psyche and the brain on immunity and disease susceptibility: a critical review." *Pschosom. Med.* 41, 1979.

7. Vermont Alternative Medicine Committee, Jan. 13, 1996, cited in *Townsend Letter for Doctors & Patients,* April 1996.

8. Culbert, *op. cit.*

9. Dossey, L., *Healing Words: the Power of Prayer and the Practice of Medicine.* New York: Harper, 1993.

10. Stone, R.B., "Cells caught in the act of communication." Newsletter, Monterey Institute for the Study of Alternative Healing Arts (MISAHA), #11, Oct.-Dec., 1995.

11. Siegel, Bernie, *Love, Medicine and Miracles.* New York: Harper and Row, 1986.

12. Northrup, C., *How to Heal Yourself from Toxic Emotions.* Potomac, MD: Phillips, 1996.

13. Zucker, M., *Cancer Warrior — Healing Through Personal Power.* Dare to Dream, Pub. 1-888-DRE-2-DRM, 1996.

Chapter XVI
HOW I GOT THAT WAY
Origins of a Conversion

In my quarter-century of practicing what many call "holistic" and "alternative" methodology against cancer, I have frequently been asked by patients how and why I "got that way."

In truth, it was more or less a gradual process, as over the years I saw more and more of the failures of conventional cancer treatments.

My skepticism began in 1955 when I served as Chief Medical Resident at Highland-Alameda County Hospital in Oakland, California.

In that capacity one of my duties was to oversee an oncology ward where some 50 cancer patients were receiving chemotherapy. As I observed and tried to care for these unfortunate and usually miserable patients, I could not help but question whether or not there was anything beneficial about the use of toxic chemicals in their treatment. Of course, I could not be too vocal about my opinions in discussing cases with my superiors, since even as chief resident I was obligated to follow the protocols laid out by the attending physicians.

It was my observation then that, almost without exception, those cancer patients were in worse condition during and after their chemotherapy than they had been before, suffering the now-well-known side effects of nausea, vomiting, malaise, anemia, secondary infections from lowered white blood cell counts, hair loss, and/or feeling just plain awful. And, of course, survivors of our "treatment" were few and far between.

I wondered, sometimes out loud, if many of these wretched souls would not be better off if they were simply left alone and allowed to die peacefully and comfortably. However, unbeknownst to me at the time, Cancer Inc. was already in place, and it would take much more than my little voice to bring about any significant changes. In all fairness, I must add that, other than the oncology experience, my days at Highland Hospital were extremely rewarding and educational.

However, of one thing I was quite certain: my practice would not include traditional oncology.

Following this learning experience, I entered the practice of internal medicine in Oakland with an older and very traditional internist. After several years of doing everything according to Hoyle and the AMA, I made the move to the Truckee-North Lake Tahoe area to join a small group of physicians, with whom I remained for about 10 years before going into solo practice in Tahoe City, California, a small town on the north shore of beautiful Lake Tahoe. This was in 1970.

In 1973, Frances Miller, one of my regular female patients, age 64 at the time, came to me with the complaint of having passed blood in the urine. She was referred to a urologist who found a very large and invasive malignant tumor in the bladder which had extended beyond the bladder wall. Two urologists had recommended complete surgical removal of the bladder along with some of the surrounding tissues which appeared to be involved. Unless this surgery was done, she was told, she would not survive more than a year, and more than likely her expectancy would be something like six months.

In spite of these dire predictions, the patient chose not to have the radical surgery but instead elected to have simple fulguration, or local removal of the tumor with electrocautery (burning). After this procedure she came to me with the question as to whether or not she should go to one of the Mexican cancer clinics to receive laetrile.

At the time I had very little knowledge of either laetrile or the cancer clinics in Tijuana, but my answer to her was something to the effect that the treatments for cancer in Mexico could hardly be any worse than those available in the US. So she was encouraged to proceed with treatment south of the border.

The clinic she chose was the Contreras Hospital in Tijuana. I asked her to find out as much about the alternative treatments available and bring what information she could back to me. This was done in due time and Frances was able to provide me with a great deal of useful information about laetrile and other non-toxic substances used by Dr. Contreras. It all seemed more logical and certainly more humane than what I had been taught were the only modalities considered to be effective in the treatment of cancer in this country.

This lady had regular cystoscopies, or "looking into the bladder" procedures over the ensuing years, with no evidence of cancer recurrence. In late 1995 she succumbed, not to cancer but to congestive heart failure, at age 86, some 21 years after her "death sentence." At the time of her death, though there had been no cystoscopies for quite a few years, there was no indication of a recurrence of her cancer.

Because of the obviously favorable results of this case, even early on, along with the scientific information I was gathering from Mexico and elsewhere, I continued to offer these alternatives to cancer patients, often in conjunction with some conventional therapy. As I gained more experience with these unconventional modalities and learned more of their effectiveness, I naturally became acquainted with other physicians and health care people with similar interests and pursuits.

The most notable of these was Dr. John Richardson, a courageous physician using laetrile and megavitamin therapy in Albany, a little town near Berkeley, California. Because of his use of the "forbidden" substance amygdalin (laetrile), Dr. Richardson had his California medical license revoked in 1976, arbitrarily and without a hearing, trial or any due process.

Shortly after this revocation, I was called by his office and asked if I would come to his rescue and assist in keeping his office open. This I agreed to do, since I considered it an important step in preserving freedom of choice for cancer patients in this country. Three other like-minded physicians also agreed to fill in, some coming from as far as 500 miles away each week. So I commuted weekly from Lake Tahoe to Albany, a distance of some 200 miles, seeing patients in Dr. Richardson's office two days of the week.

The four of us managed to keep Dr. Richardson's office open and very busy for the next four years. As you can well imagine, all of this activity did not go unnoticed by the regulators of doctors, then known in California as the Board of Medical Quality Assurance, or BMQA, the same folks who had summarily revoked Dr. Richardson's license for the use of laetrile and other "crimes." Since we were continuing the same type of activity, and since regulators are always compelled to regulate, their next target was — no surprise — me, of course.

Over those four years I was subjected to many court appearances, including two "trials" conducted by the State of California at the behest of the BMQA. Each lasted several weeks, and each was presided over by an "administrative law judge" hired by the state for the purpose of suspending, revoking or by one manner or another disabling my license to practice medicine in California.

Although it was known by all concerned that these attacks on my license were because of laetrile and my unorthodox approach to the treatment of cancer, the state chose not to attack me directly over these issues. This could possibly have been due to the fact that at all times I had been in compliance with the law, or what sufficed for law in those days — namely, the "affidavit system" set up by a federal judge which allowed patients to legally receive laetrile.

Instead of attacking me on this front, the BMQA used one of its favorite avenues (a back road in this case) — the charge of "over-prescribing narcotics."

My first knowledge of this came to me by way of the local newspaper, on the front page of which was a headline reading "Warrant Issued for Doctor's Arrest," under which read "Physician Charged With 23 Felonies." To my horror, the article was about me! I had not been issued a warrant or any other notification that I was wanted by anybody.

Calling my attorney immediately, I was able to avoid arrest by going to the local sheriff's office and entering a plea. The state operatives had presented a warrant to the Placer County Sheriff's Office but had told the sheriff's deputies not to act upon it because they, members of BMQA, wanted to make the arrest themselves. (This, by the way, occurred on a Friday, and, as I learned later, it is frequently the modus operandi of the state operatives to make their arrests late on Friday nights, with TV cameras present, to achieve the highest level of humiliation.) Also with the weekend coming up, bail is, of course, difficult if not impossible, and the victim must "sit it out" in jail at least until the following Monday.

The 23 felonies, as it turned out, represented 23 individual prescriptions, all legally and justifiably written. The state agency later admitted in court that none of these was an actual felony and it had "made a mistake." Of course, the newspaper, having perpetuated this little "mistake," never made a retraction, correction, or acknowledgment of error. So the damage was done, and my reputation (which was and is my livelihood) had been permanently impaired. Nevertheless the "trial" proceeded as scheduled.

The allegedly offending prescriptions involved those of four patients, all with serious and painful conditions, but strangely none suffering from cancer. Most notable of the patients chosen by BMQA to use in its attack was a young man with Buerger's disease, which is a painful condition affecting the blood supply to the extremities.

This unfortunate man had had some 40 amputations in the course of his lifelong affliction because of gangrene, which would affect a portion of a finger or toe at a time until finally his arms had been amputated at the mid-forearm and his legs were off at the hips. He had received huge quantities of narcotic pain-relievers from University of California hospitals where most of the amputations had been carried out. I had been prescribing the same medications to him, actually in lower doses than had been prescribed by the University of California-San Francisco (UCSF).

Prior to the notification of the warrant, I had been visited in my office by two state BMQA agents demanding, among other things, the records on the above patient. They also ordered me to stop prescribing narcotics to this pathetic figure of a man in constant pain, with no arms or legs, unable to care for himself.

I was crudely and rudely threatened with license revocation if I did not comply with this order. I reluctantly complied, since I had seen what this agency could do and had done to competent and honorable physicians such as Dr. Richardson, and since I felt that this patient could obtain his medication elsewhere, such as the University of California medical departments in San Francisco or Davis, as he had done before.

What I did not know at the time was that these same agents had "visited" some of the patient's other physicians and threatened them as well.

Such threats and demands on the part of government agents are not only illegal but outside their jurisdiction or area of authority, which places them as individuals in a legally vulnerable position.

Within a month of being denied his legal prescriptions, the patient died, no doubt painfully, because on the day of his death he had "shot up" a bag of street heroin in a desperate attempt to relieve his pain. Interestingly, and probably not coincidentally, my "warrant" was issued within a short time of this patient's demise. Did they wait for the man to die, knowing that the appearance of an armless and legless man would bring out a lot of sympathy in a courtroom? We can only guess.

The trial was conducted in Tahoe City, a master stroke by my very competent attorney, Bob Maddox. Because the proceedings were held in my home town and because I was fortunate to have an abundance of local support, the courtroom was packed with my supporters and patients. This appeared to influence the judge favorably.

However, at one point the entire audience was ejected because its support of me had become too vociferous. One doctor, testifying for the state, was asked how he would deal with the medical addiction of the patient in question. His reply was, "I would just get him hooked on other drugs." This inane remark brought down the house and spurred the eviction.

Another interesting highlight was that a review of all the narcotic prescriptions to all of the pharmacies in the area revealed that I was the "low man on the totem pole." I had prescribed fewer narcotics than any other physician in the area over the previous year! This fact alone speaks volumes about the motivation and the code of ethics of the BMQA and the State of California.

Mine is not an isolated case. Certain doctors are targeted for elimination, often for their unorthodox beliefs and approaches to medical care, especially in the area of cancer.

The targeting is done by a panel of the AMA called the "Committee on Quackery," and the implementation of this is carried out by the FDA, which in turn applies the pressure on the state licensing agencies to put the selected doctor out of business. The Mafia-like committee of the AMA has compiled a "hit list" of doctors marked for extinction, and I am known to be on the list, having hired a private investigator to gather this and other information. (One of the first principles of warfare is to "know your enemy.")

The "administrative law judge," hostile at first, eventually could see that no crime had been committed, and that I had been simply trying to render the most humane and merciful care to the multiple amputee as well as to the other patients. Consequently the decision was in my favor, for the most part.

My license was not revoked or suspended, but a minor technical violation was found regarding narcotic prescriptions, having to do with patients taking their prescriptions across state lines to have them filled.

Being close to the state line, it had been customary and acceptable for some California patients living near the border to fill their prescriptions at a pharmacy in Crystal Bay, Nevada, which is just across the California-Nevada state line. This I had personally cleared with the heads of the boards of pharmacy of both states several years before the various charges were leveled against me.

Telephone prescriptions were also considered acceptable, and this was being done by most, if not all, of the physicians in the area.

Nevertheless, the judge and the state apparently had to save face and find me guilty of something. My narcotic writing privilege was suspended for a few months, but this was not a serious impairment since I had never written a lot of prescriptions for controlled substances anyway and because I could refer patients needing narcotic medications to nearby colleagues. This privilege was reinstated after a few months, and I thought all was (almost) well.

The State of California, in particular the licensing board, angered over failure to put me out of business, initiated another action about two years after the first unsuccessful attack.

The second assault was almost a carbon copy of the first. Again the issue was over-prescribing narcotics, and again just as phony. The selective detectives from the BMQA had been able to find patients — this time only two — to whom I had prescribed narcotics. The state sleuths had uncovered or manufactured another reprehensible crime — over-prescribing controlled substances.

Again the trial was held in my home territory, and again the town turned out in substantial numbers in my support. Again the state demonstrated that it had no case, and again it failed to find sufficient grounds to suspend or revoke my license. But again, the damage was done to my psyche, my physical well-being, and of course to my pocketbook.

Not content with this outcome, however, the state agents then launched a third attack, again using their favorite MO, the over-prescribing caper. You would think they might have used a little more imagination.

By this time I was definitely getting the feeling that I was being harassed, selectively persecuted and prosecuted. Against my lawyer's (by this time a different lawyer in the same firm) advice, I decided to take the initiative and go on the offensive.

With the help of a good paralegal, I drew up a document pointing out that the board was now engaging in harassment and was exceeding its jurisdiction, citing legal precedents to affirm this position.

I called for and was granted a meeting with the BMQA board in Sacramento, and a copy of this document was presented to each member of the board. I then gave a brief presentation of my position and stated that if the board continued to pursue what I considered to be harassment and activity beyond their authority, I would take legal action against each of them individually.

They responded by saying that they would "take this under advisement" and would advise me as to their decision. About three weeks later I received a letter from the board saying that they had decided not to pursue the action. Needless to say, I was elated and greatly relieved not to have to go through another expensive and exhausting trial along with the inevitable adverse publicity. Of course, I wondered if, by taking this course of action in the first place, I could have avoided the agony and expense of both of the previous trials.

I wondered also why the lawyers had been so opposed to an action so obviously effective. This was perhaps the biggest "eye-opener" of the whole experience. With all due respect to the lawyers, who did an excellent job in this case, all attorneys are "officers of the court" and are thus obligated to follow specific procedures and to stay within certain limitations.

The "pro se" or "pro per" litigant, acting as his own lawyer, is not bound by the same restrictions. This is not to say that we do not need lawyers, since most of us do not have the time or the expertise to follow the intricacies of law and procedure. But there are certain situations, as in confronting a government agency, in which lawyers can be part of the problem.

By the time the threat of a third trial loomed into view, I had come to the realization that some very powerful people wanted me out of the way, or at the very least, out of the State of California. (Some of us are slower to learn than others.)

Actually I had realized this to some degree earlier, having witnessed the attack on Dr. Richardson and others. But I was not ready to surrender until this "last straw" brought me to the realization that the BMQA and other government agencies, with unlimited funds (the taxpayers'), would keep coming after me until I was exhausted in mind, body, spirit, and resources.

Hence, in 1980 I made the decision to move to Nevada, where laws regarding medical choices were more tolerant. These included a law legalizing laetrile which I, along with co-author Mike Culbert, had previously helped to get passed by the Nevada Legislature.

Several years before, anticipating this exigency, I had also obtained a Nevada medical license. Fortunately, the move was not a long one.

About 15 miles from Tahoe City, eastward along Lake Tahoe's north shore, lay Incline Village, just across the state line into Nevada. This seemed to be a natural destination, so here I settled down to continue to pursue what I considered to be my right to practice medicine, not according to orthodoxy but according to my conscience, still concentrating on better and safer methods of dealing with cancer and other degenerative diseases. My patients continued to fare much better, for the most part, than those limiting their care to conventional treatments.

Shortly after this move, the State of California passed a draconian law making it a felony for a physician to administer any substance or procedure to a cancer patient other than the "big three" — chemotherapy, radiation and surgery. Consequently, had I remained in California, and had I continued my non-traditional methods, I might very well have gone to jail for my efforts.

Excellence in medicine flourishes in the free marketplace of ideas, unfettered by special interests such as the pharmaceutical industry. New and different concepts must be allowed and encouraged in order for true progress to be made. Unfortunately for patients in this country, and for mankind in general, progress in the treatment of cancer and the other so-called "degenerative diseases" has moved at a snail's pace. (Maybe more like an anvil's.)

This is remarkable in light of the fact that our diagnostic capabilities have advanced so rapidly. Establishment medicine has developed many marvelous gadgets for locating tumors, such as the CT Scanner, MRI, PET scan and the like, with new developments appearing almost daily. But these new inventions and devices seem to be largely confined to the area of diagnosis.

Orthodox *treatment* methods have remained relatively unchanged over the last 50 or 60 years, at least in the field of cancer.

It should be mentioned, of course, that many of the amazing techniques of modern surgery do not seem to be so restricted by orthodoxy, and are to be admired on the same level as the new diagnostic procedures. It is more the basic premises of medical therapy, the apparent abandonment of the basic premise of "do no harm," and the disdain shown toward prevention that need to be seriously re-examined by mainstream or orthodox medicine.

Incidentally, if we look up the word *orthodox* in the dictionary, we find that it is derived from the Greek word *orthodoxos,* which means "having the right opinion," or adhering to traditional or commonly accepted beliefs. Believing that the earth was flat was once the accepted view and the "right opinion."

One of the factors that was highly influential, in a negative way, in contributing to my conversion away from the mainstream and into alternative or complementary care of cancer patients has been the obvious bias which prevails in the traditional medical journals.

As a conventional practicing physician I received around 40 different medical journals every month — most of them free, of course.

Even before my conversion, I wouldn't actually *pay* for all that material, most of which was advertising.

It should be apparent to even the most orthodox physician that the primary purveyor of medical information in this country is the pharmaceutical industry. Big, splashy, multicolored ads dominate its journals, almost to the exclusion of useful information. Such information as one might find in these publications is skewed in favor of drug therapy.

Of course, I did not take any surgical journals, which, from the few I have seen, contain more technical and useful information, with less of the pro-drug bias. But always the direction of flow is mainstream. Never have I seen a meaningful or positive article on diet or nutritional influences on disease in a conventional journal. For this kind of information one must turn to those publications which are outside the mainstream, a partial list of which is provided at the end of this chapter.

What is obviously needed in this scenario is to break down the barriers erected by the establishment which prevent the free flow of information to physicians. There is much scientifically valid work which has been systematically excluded from mainstream literature. Younger physicians, in particular, need to have access to all aspects of medicine, mainstream and otherwise.

Back in the middle ages, it was the Church that was the protector of orthodoxy or predominant doctrine. Today the role has been taken over by bureaucratic and collectivist-oriented institutions, of which the universities and government are unfortunately examples.

The FDA, as one example, imposes the predominant doctrine of drug-oriented medicine by protecting the pharmaceutical industry. One of the many ways that it does this is by making stricter and stricter limitations on the use and availability of natural substances and methodologies. The attack on my license was but one of many such attacks across the country.

As noted by Gustave Le Bon, the intelligent behavior of a group adheres to entirely different laws from that of the individual. The herd can proceed only as fast as its slowest member. The individual, without collectivist restraints, may acquire as much knowledge and achieve whatever levels of accomplishment his or her intelligence, talent and industry will permit.

When minds are not trapped in the cage of orthodoxy, great achievements are not only possible, but inevitable. Medicine and the pursuit of medical knowledge should be free and unfettered, regulation being directed primarily toward the safety of patients. Effectiveness of modalities would then be determined by the marketplace and the free exchange of ideas, not by groups of bureaucrats or statisticians who have little practical knowledge of how medical care and medicines actually work.

The arrogance of the medical establishment is becoming more and more apparent in the field of cancer, as the public is assured repeatedly that "these are the only methods that work," referring, of course, to chemotherapy, radiation, and surgery.

More and more Americans are developing a healthy skepticism toward this "official opinion," as they find that in fact these highly touted methods do *not* work. Oncologists and other traditional practitioners are ethically, and in some states, legally, bound to inform patients as to all treatment options available to them.

Only in very rare instances does this informing include any of the alternative methods, most physicians still being bound by official opinion and limited to the "cut, burn, and poison" mentality.

One of the refreshing exceptions to this has been my association with an outstanding oncologist, Dr. James Forsythe, who has had the vision and the courage to explore — and even utilize — alternatives in his practice, along with conventional chemotherapy. I have been privileged to participate in the care of many of his patients and vice-versa. Together we have found, quite consistently, that immune support and proper supplementation greatly reduce — and frequently eliminate altogether — the drastic side effects of chemotherapy.

We have also found that patients usually respond better to chemotherapy while receiving such supplementation. Dr. Forsythe has pursued the study of alternative methods even to the extent that he has obtained a license in homeopathy, which has to be a first among board-certified oncologists. Of course, as one might expect, this activity has drawn fire from the licensing board and from his oncological colleagues.

Speaking of homeopathy, one of the steps in my conversion was to obtain a license in this discipline, which I did in 1983 when a law was passed in Nevada establishing this as a legal entity and establishing a Board of Homeopathic Medical Examiners.

I was appointed by then Governor (now Senator) Richard Bryan to serve on this board in the state and was its first vice president. My homeopathic license was the second such issued in the state, the first being awarded to Board President Fuller Royal MD, HMD. The function of the homeopathic board, as with the allopathic board, is to regulate the issuance of licenses, establish and maintain high standards of practice in the field of homeopathy, and to discipline, when necessary, any physician not maintaining those standards.

The "bottom line" of any conversion to alternative methods is that the right of the individual to exercise his or her freedom of choice in medical care must not be violated by government or anybody else. It is the primary goal of government to protect and defend these rights rather than to attack them, as is sadly the case today. Serious inquiry must be made into natural alternatives to drug-oriented medicine, which is what this book is all about.

PARTIAL LIST OF ALTERNATIVE PUBLICATIONS

Alternative Medicine Digest.
Future Medicine Publishing, Inc.
1640 Tiburon Blvd., Suite 2
Tiburon, CA 94920

Alternative Therapies in Health and Medicine
InnoVision Communications
101 Columbia, Aliso Viejo, CA 92656

Townsend Letter for Doctors and Patients
911 Tyler St. Port Townsend, WA 98368

The Journal of Alternative and Complementary Therapies
Mary Ann Liebert, Inc.
2 Madison Ave., Larchmont, NY 10538

Health and Healing
Julian Whitaker, MD
Phillips Publishing
7811 Montrose Rd., Potomac, MD 20854

Journal of Advancement in Medicine
ACAM, American College of Advancement in Medicine
Human Sciences Press, Inc.
233 Spring St., NY, NY 10013

Alternatives — For the Health Conscious Individual
Dr. David Williams
Mountain Home Publishing
2700 Cummings Lane, Kerrville, TX 78028

Journal of Longevity Research
Health Quest Publications
316 California Avenue
Reno, NV 89509

The Choice
Committee for Freedom of Choice in Medicine, Inc.
1180 Walnut Avenue
Chula Vista, CA 91911

Naturally Well. Healing with the Power of Nature
Dr. Marcus Laux
Phillips Publishing Inc.
7811 Montrose Rd., Potomac, MD 20854

The Mindell Letter
Dr. Earl Mindell
Phillips Publishing, Inc.
7811 Montrose Road, Potomac, MD 20854

Health and Longevity
Robert D. Willix Jr., MD
105 West Monument St.
P.O. Box 17477
Baltimore, MD 21298

Health Revelations
Dr. Robert Atkins
P.O. Box 17097
Baltimore, MD 21298

Health Freedom News
National Health Federation
Monrovia, CA

Chapter XVII
HOW MEDICINE GOT THAT WAY:
A Paradigm in Transformation

As I began my conversion to a new way of medical thinking, it did not take me too long to realize I was actually treading on well-trod ground:

A return to what many call the "holistic" concept of seeing man as a union of mind, spirit *and* body, with the parallel realization that to treat only one part of this triad without addressing the other two is inadequate medicine at best, a catastrophe at worst.

In fact, virtually all of medicine, however defined, in one or more ways held to the holistic concept — or, as modern psychologists prefer, *paradigm,* or organized thought system — as late as the middle of the nineteenth century.

My co-author has labored over the serpentine history of medical thought (*Medical Armageddon*) to which I refer readers who seek a detailed historical study of its evolution.(1) A few points loom of significance and should be understood by anyone who seeks to answer the question, "How *did* medicine get that way?"

MEDICINE IS AN ART, NOT A SCIENCE

Even as late as this century, practitioners of medicine (as variously defined) normally realized they were involved in "the medical arts," despite an economic/industrial rush to define the corpus of medicine as a *science*, to be held hostage to a rigid set of beliefs about the nature of science as primarily postulated by philosophers and innovative observers — particularly Rene Descartes (1596-1650) and Sir Isaac Newton (1642-1727).

The advent (described below) of "the germ theory of disease" in the 19th century did much to advance the notion that there was such a thing as "medical science."

But from time immemorial the healer or physician — at least up to the 19th century — had been as interested in the emotional/mental condition of the patient, and all the subtleties of his physical self, as he was in the actual process of a disease condition. The gathering of data on the total person's internal, external and even emotional/spiritual environment — usually called the "terrain" in the 19th century — was both empirical and intuitive, which is to say "non-scientific" in the strictest sense.

But, however many aspects of science (guaranteed reproducibility of outcomes, known mechanical aspects of the body and the healing process, etc.) as may exist in medicine, it remains — as *healing* — far more an art-form than a science. Dissenters agree: the phrase "scientific medicine" is a contradiction in terms.

MEDICINE TAKES MANY FORMS

The "healing arts" — as they were once more properly known — over time took many forms.

No one seriously argues that the most ancient form of medicine was the laying on of hands (religious ritual), swiftly followed by the advent of finding useful medicinal plants (herbs), animal secretions and minerals as curative elements.[2]

By the nineteenth century in the United States it was widely understood that there were many forms of medicine.

The more prominent were botanical medicine, bone-setting, eclecticism (borrowing from several schools), followers of Sylvester Graham, Christian Science and the titans which finally fought for dominance over all others — homeopathy and allopathy.

As late as the final decade of the 20th century, it is difficult to find an American who is really cognizant of the latter two words, and almost nobody is taught in public schools just what an "allopath" is.

Yet "allopath" appears in all foreign languages of consequence and it is generally understood in them that "allopathy" usually refers in general to the treatment of diseases by "contraries" or "opposites" — that is, drugs, surgery, radiation, the accouterments of what more normally is called in the USA "standard" or even "scientific" medicine.

The term was better known in the America of the 19th century because it was opposed by an opposite doctrine — homeopathy, the treating of diseases by "similars," which laid every bit as much claim to being "scientific" as did the drug-dispensing allopaths.

Homeopathy, essentially utilizing minuscule dilutions of (mostly) plant-derived material "proved" against specific symptoms, had, by the middle of the last century, become by far the major adversary of surgically and drug-oriented allopathic medicine. Homeopathy cost less, often cured more, and its practitioners were more influential and often traveled in higher social circles than the allopaths.(3)

It was the coming of the "germ theory of disease," as championed in Europe by Koch and Pasteur, which represented the most important philosophical fork in the road for Western medicine:

The discovery that "germs" or "microbes" seemed to cause many diseases led to a new paradigm: namely, that health is the absence of disease and that disease, perhaps *all* disease, is caused by "germs," variously to be defined as microbes, parasites, bacteria, and viruses.

The coming of the germ theory virtually disabled French traditional medical teaching, at the time the Western international standard of medical thought and progress. It meant that, after all, it was the *germ,* not the "terrain," which should be medicine's prime concern.

We now know, of course, and from different observers, that on his deathbed Louis Pasteur confessed defeat in his ideological struggle with Claude Bernard: "Bernard was right: the germ is nothing, the terrain is everything."(4)

It is not much of a leap in logic to understand how neatly allopathic theory fitted the market demands of the synthetic drug industry, which incubated during the American Civil War but reached far greater dimensions early in the present century.

By the time allopathy, supported by the drug industry, was grinding homeopathy almost out of existence, the former was being challenged by naturopathy (a European import) and by osteopathy, which it eventually co-opted. It would, much later, be challenged on a grand scale by chiropractic.

In 1908, two highly influential and extremely wealthy men, John D. Rockefeller and Andrew Carnegie, both already deeply involved in chemical and drug interests, set out to "reform" medical education in America. To this end, they commissioned Abraham Flexner to conduct a survey of all the medical schools, many of which were actually badly in need of upgrading at the time.

Some medical degrees could be obtained by mail-order and many could be acquired with minimal training. Medical schools were underfunded and understaffed. So the time was ripe for reform, and these opportunists were quick to seize the opportunity. The result of this effort was the "Flexner Report" which recommended the strengthening of courses in *pharmacology* and the establishment of research, which was primarily drug-oriented, in all medical schools deemed by them to be "qualified."

While the Flexner Report undoubtedly performed a needed service at the time, the ultimate effect was the conversion of US medical schools from teaching mostly natural and non-toxic modalities to promoting drug-oriented medical disciplines. This "report" was backed by enormous financial clout, since the architects of this scheme held the purse strings to medical education through their immensely wealthy foundations.

Subsequent events revealed the ulterior motives of the designers. Following the report, Rockefeller and Carnegie began to shower many millions of dollars on the medical schools which were willing to make this conversion. The rest gradually died on the vine, and with them their principal disciplines such as homeopathy and naturopathy.(5,6)

By the second decade of this century, the industrial combination of synthetic drugs, medical licensure, medical research funds, medical schools, donations from enormously wealthy families with at times hidden socio/political agendas, had fused into what is today "standard" or "scientific" medicine.

The word *allopathy* nowhere commonly appears, of course, because to use it might lead the laity into the realization that if there is "allopathic medicine " then in fact there might be other kinds of healing arts which have an equal right to be called "medicine." Because there are.

Allopathy — now enshrined in the American Medical Association, formed in the 1840s primarily to thwart homeopathy, and which should more ethically have called itself the American Allopathic Medical Association — has co-opted the words "medicine," "physician" and "doctor" almost entirely in American English usage.

Allopathy's primary tenets — and the reasons for its present free-fall into increasing disrepute — remain these:

• Understanding the germ or pathogen is more important than understanding the terrain of the "host," or patient.

• Health is the absence of disease, and disease is caused by germs.

• Man is a mass of physical parts, a kind of perpetual-motion machine in a physical universe.

• The mental/spiritual and physical aspects of man are separate and distinct.

• Scientific medicine is the understanding and management of each part and each function of each physical part of the body (hence, medical specialties abound).

• Each disease condition is best treated by one "contrary" at a time (monopharmacy).

It just happens that this line of thinking has a lot going for it in terms of infectious, single-cause bacterial and parasitical diseases, against which allopathy has scored its most impressive victories.

And, in terms of "trauma" medicine, the rescue of accident victims at death's door, the saving of a leg, the resuscitation of a flagging heart, allopathy has achieved numerous marvels and successes which cannot be ignored and should never be underestimated.

Yet in at least temporarily conquering many of the bacterial infectious diseases of old and providing mechanical successes in advanced trauma medicine, allopathy — by abandoning the holistic paradigm — is, by itself, an inadequate performer against the major disease challenges of the civilized Western world.

CHRONIC DISEASE HAS ALTERED THE PARADIGM

The very nature of allopathy renders it conceptually unable to grasp the single most important element in the modern chronic diseases which now plague the West:

Multifactoriality.

This concept holds that there are multiple causes of chronic disease, immune dysregulations, and the like, and that there are multiple treatments for the same. The idea of one-drug, one-disease becomes a useless "magic bullet" notion when arrayed, for example, against cancer, the many conditions called "heart disease," diabetes, environmental disease, the ever-growing list of immunological disturbances ranging from autoimmune diseases to all aspects of AIDS, the lengthening list of pediatric and geriatric conditions, a raft of musculoneurological disorders, and — of course— even the common cold.

The history of modern medicine in America has been a virtual tradeoff:

As infectious diseases of old succumbed to allopathic methods of treatment and prevention (antibiotics, vaccines, immunizations, etc.), chronic diseases loomed as the new mass killers, sweeping relentlessly through ever broader sectors of the "civilized" population. As the numbers — in incidence, in fatalities, in untold, lingering suffering — have continued, people in general, and many doctors in particular, have looked for a better way.

CANCER IS THE GREAT LEVELER

The widespread presence of cancer in the Western world has thus been the great leveler and the provoker of new thought in medicine.

It is the allopathic thought-process, so rooted in the 17th century, which still wishes to see cancer as multiple kinds of tumors, each with a different "cause," each needing a different "treatment," rather than as a multifactorial malignant process which involves the triad of mind, body and spirit.

The idea that cancer, as a disease, whether "caused" by viruses, aberrant genes, or something else, can be burned away, poisoned out or surgically removed, is entirely allopathic — and, most of the time, entirely inadequate. Continual allegiance to the allopathic paradigm, and the multiple industries which nourish it, is the central reason for the essential failure of Cancer Inc.

At the present time, metastatic cancer — malignancy spread from one site to another — has an abysmally low "cure" rate, as we have seen (*see Chapter III*). The hideous new calamity before the Western world, AIDS, so far has no "cure" at all. And about a quarter of AIDS is, by definition, cancer.

With *all* of AIDS and *most* of metastatic cancer, and virtually *all* of the autoimmune diseases now classed as "incurable," there can be no wonder why a medical revolution is breaking out — and why I joined it.

INTEGRATIVE MEDICINE IS MODERN-DAY HOLISM

Those of us in this revolution realize that we are in effect rediscovering the ancient, virtually universal concept of holism.

But many of us also realize that this is not a reaction of bringing back the past to save the future — we wish to integrate into medicine *all* forms of legitimate healing — indeed, anything that "works."

This means that, while we will continue to place ever-growing importance on nutrition, attitudes and natural therapies, we will not fail to use *any* practice or technique which fulfills the Hippocratic mandate in medicine: save lives, reduce suffering. And, above all, do no harm. We do not seek to replace or eliminate any of the good that exists in modern medicine.

In this new and integrative model, allopathic medicine has a definite and important role.

The joining of forces between drug-centered allopathic medicine, natural therapies and breakthrough diagnostics will eventually bring victory over cancer, as some of the cases in this book clearly show.

More importantly, it will be the keystone of the medicine of the 21st century — the promotion of health.

REFERENCES

1. Culbert, M.L., *Medical Armageddon.* San Diego: C and C Communications, 1995.
2. "Faith and the Human Touch." In *Powers of Healing.* New York: Life-Time Books, 1989.
3. Coulter, H.L., *Divided Legacy: The Conflict between Homoeopathy and the American Medical Association.* Richmond, CA: North Atlantic Books, 1973.
4. Ornstein, Robert, and Sobel, David, *The Healing Brain.* New York: Simon and Schuster, 1987.
5. Culbert, M.L., *op. cit.*
6. Griffin, G.E., *World Without Cancer.* Westlake Village, CA: American Media, 1974.

Chapter XVIII
SUPPRESSION OF ALTERNATIVES

WHAT'S GOING ON HERE?

Throughout this book we have seen many instances of suppression of safe, reasonable and viable alternative methods of treatment of a hitherto incurable disease. Such suppression is not a new phenomenon in the field of medicine, but actually can be found throughout much of its history.

In the mid-1800s, when many new mothers were dying of puerperasl sepsis or blood stream infection following childbirth, an observant and innovative Australian physician, Dr. Ignasz Semmelweis, suggested that doctors simply wash hands before delivering babies. For this "radical" view -- which of course later proved to be correct — this good and conscientious physician was ridiculed, persecuted and ostracized by his colleagues to the point that he was driven insane (or at least regarded as insane) and taken to a mental institution where he eventually died.

The "mainstream" doctors of that time apparently could not stand the thought that they themselves might actually be causing the many post-partum infections which were then so often leading to suffering and death.

In England another physician named Joseph Lister was similarly attacked by the establishment physicians of his day for suggesting that the many post-surgical infections of that time might be avoided if the surgeons would use sterile techniques. Many of the procedures suggested by Lister are used to this day in maintaining sterility in operating rooms in this country and throughout the world.

In our country, another medical pioneer with impeccable credentials, Dr. William Koch, ran afoul of the medical establishment in a somewhat different way. This physician had made significant contributions to the world's scientific knowledge about the parathyroid glands. These tiny glands, which regulate calcium metabolism and are situated right next to the thyroid gland, were once unwittingly removed by surgeons in the course of thyroidectomy. Death would frequently ensue from tetany, a type of convulsion due to the loss of regulation of calcium by the parthyroids. Koch's work on this subject led to preservation of the parathyroids during surgery and the saving of many lives.

The *Journal of the American Medical Association* published the work of this innovative physician in 1913 with a highly complimentary editorial. Six years later in the same journal he was scornfully branded as a fraud and a quack. What had taken place in this short time to bring about such a drastic reversal of editorial attitude was Dr. Koch's entering upon the forbidden field of cancer. He had brought forth the concept that cancer results from insuffering oxidation or inadequate consumption of oxygen, along with inadequate removal of toxins from the body, concepts which he taught at Wayne University in Michigan from 1914 to 1919.

When Koch then developed a treatment for cancer based upon his observations, he was severely reprimanded by the Wayne County Medical Society as well as the AMA and the rest of the medical establishment. Even though he was dragged over the coals by his own profession, Koch was highly praised in the halls of congress for his work. Nevertheless he was prosecuted by the FDA in two trials in the 1940s in which the government attacked his oxidation theory of treating cancer. The relentless attack continued until the agency was able to obtain a permanent injunction against his work in 1950, driving him to ruin and exile in Brazil.

At no point in this battle were his theories ever disproved or his treatment shown to be ineffective. His treatment with *Glyoxylide* is used to this day in various parts of the world and his theories have withstood the test of time, but remains on the fringe and far from acceptance by mainstream medicine. Koch's story is further evidence of the arbitrary and dominating nature of Cancer Inc. and its allies in the FDA, who somehow "have their way" regardless of what anybody else thinks, including the US Congress.

There are many similar cases of this bias in recent times, including that of the late Linus Pauling, who remained a favorite of officialdom and sanctioned media until he took on the forces of the cancer establishment. (*see Chapter VII*) When Pauling had the audacity to contend that vitamin C might be of help in the care of cancer, he was relegated to the trash heap of official opinion.

In centuries past, this resistance to change in medicine might variously be attributed to arrogance, ignorance, fear of the unknown, or some kind of fragile professional egotism. But the present-day version of this obstinacy has taken on a different and more malignant character, becoming more pervasive, more aggressive and more organized, particularly in the field of cancer. Here the "Establishment" seems to be more closed-minded and intolerant than in any other branch of medicine, going to extraordinary lengths to force its uncompromising point of view on those whose ideas may differ from those of the "consensus."

Today, a prime example of this is the case of Stanislaw Burzyznski, MD, PhD, who is discussed elsewhere in this book (Chapter VX). As we have noted, this physician/biochemist had emigrated from his native Poland to escape the communist oppression which had so severely affected him and his work, only to find similar persecution in the United States.

For many years, Dr. Burzynski did extensive clinical research into certain peptides or amino acid complexes found in human urine. These he now calls "Antineoplastons" because of their inhibiting effect on cancer cells (also called neoplastic cells). He found that the peptides had the capacity to normalize cells that were defective or which were undergoing degeneration (in other words turning into cancer cells.) He also found that these natural body substances were part of the human defense system in what he regarded as a "parallel defense system."

This highly competent and brilliant physician/scientist has treated thousands of cancer patients in his Houston clinic, called the Burzynski Research Institute or BRI. Many of his results have been very successful, and some spectacularly so.

The Cancer Establishment, true to form and remaining intolerant of any ideas other than its own, launched an unmerciful and unrelenting attack on this courageous physician. On at least three occasions over the past dozen years the FDA had attempted to obtain Grand Jury Indictments against Dr. Burzynski. Each of these attempts had failed because of lack of convincing evidence. On the fourth try, by picking its own Grand Jury and providing it with one-sided information, the federal agency was finally able to "procure" an indictment.

For years, the FDA, along with local enforcement agencies, has conducted numerous raids on the Burzynski clinic, seizing patients records and other documents confirming the effectiveness of the antineoplastons. Dr. Burzynski has endured many court battles, and through it all has managed to keep his clinic open, although its survival has been tenuous at times. As of this writing, and despite a mistrial in the government's main case against him, it was not at all evident that the harassment was over.

The most spectacular results from the use of the Antineoplastons have been with brain tumors, especially those occurring in children. This, of course, has been an area in which conventional oncology has been particularly unsuccessful. Government agents, acting as though they were licensed to practice medicine, have even gone so far as to force the withholding of this life-saving medicine from patients, including children whose brain tumors had literally vanished as a result of Dr. Burzynski's peptide preparations. There have been several documented cases in which brain tumors have reappeared in children whose medication had been forcibly withheld by the FDA under the direction of Commissioner David Kessler. (Kessler resigned in December 1996.)

How could anyone, or any group, be so heartless as to withhold, or cause to be withheld, medication or material that is obviously keeping patients alive? This seems especially unconscionable when those patients are children, and when the withholder is an agency of the US government.

The "bottom line" of all this is that government at any level, whether it be federal, state or other jurisdiction, has no right to interfere with the doctor-patient relationship or to intervene in medical decisions mutually arrived at between physician and patient. This should especially hold true in cases where the patient is suffering from a fatal illness for which orthodox medicine has no cure. When a federal agency deprives a terminal patient of his or her freedom of choice as to treatment modality, that agency then undermines the hope and morale of that patient, who already has a serious morale problem.

Not content with the harassment of Dr. Burzynski and his patients, the medicrats have prevailed upon insurance companies to refuse to pay for this type of care, and they have even brought in the State of Texas to apply still more bureaucratic pressure upon BRI. This has become typical of the seemingly irrational behavior of all levels of government toward what they obviously consider a serious threat to Cancer Inc.

Usually, the media faithfully line up with the governmental/pharmaceutical/industrial axis in such cases -- but a strange thing happened in the Burzynski case:

Overkill boomeranged.

As the plight of "Dr. B" was consistently aired in the press and over television, and as case after case of his patients being denied life-saving treatments by the government's harassment of their physician came to light, it was the FDA and Cancer Inc. that started looking more and more like monsters, while the Polish emigre quietly reached folk-hero status.

There are many other cases of selective persecution which have been well documented elsewhere, including *Medical Armageddon* by co-author Culbert, previously referred to. All of these cases tell basically the same story -- a consistent pattern of selective harassment, persecution, and prosecution of physicians and other professionals who have dared to deviate from the accepted "norm" in the care of cancer. It is becoming more and more apparent that Cancer Inc. cannot tolerate competition and shows no sign of relinquishing its exclusive control over the treatment of cancer, this control being zealously protected by the federal government.

For many years, I have struggled with the questions that naturally arise from all of this. How could such suppression happen in a free country? Don't people realize that many thousands of lives -- actually millions as these policies are extended over many years -- are at stake? Why would such arrogant and tyrannical behavior on the part of a government agency be allowed by legislators supposedly responsive to the will of the people? Who is responsible for this apparently inhumane disregard for the hundreds of thousands of Americans suffering and dying of cancer?

For a time I attributed this obviously callous attitude to colossal greed on the part of the pharmaceutical giants and all of their affiliates in the industry, and this is obviously a major element. However, if avarice were the sole motivating factor, why would government agencies at all levels provide the enforcement muscle to perpetuate such outrageous crimes against humanity as the acts against Dr. Burzynski and his patients? After all, government agents are salaried and are thus paid just the same whether they commit these atrocities or not, this being true of their superiors on up the line as well. It seems clear that there is more at work here than greed alone, even taking into consideration the likelihood of payoff in some instances.

The history of the Food and Drug Administration (FDA) is a story of a good idea gone bad. The original intent of the first Food and Drug Act of 1906 was to protect the consumer by requiring that a list of ingredients be included on all packages of medicines, among other aspects of the act. The agency remained relatively small and the law remained, for the most part, favorable to the public interest for many years.

In 1938, additional authority was given the agency with the passage of the Food, Drug and Cosmetic Act (FDCA) which imposed the requirement of demonstrated safety on all new drugs. While this was a commendable goal, this step imposed substantial new financial requirements for the development of new drugs. This act also solidified the monopoly of allopathic medicine by establishing that only the MD physician had the right to prescribe medications.

The next major increase in power granted the FDA came in 1962, following the Thalidomide disaster in Europe, which resulted in many deformed babies from a hastily approved drug. The consequences of this were the Kefauver amendments to the FDCA, requiring that a drug be proven *effective* as well as safe. Ironically, the excuse for these new requirements was the Thalidomide scandal which had nothing to do with effectiveness but rather with *safety*, which was already covered by the law prior to the 1962 amendments. All of this, of course, resulted in much more extensive regulation being required for the approval of new drugs, further escalating the costs of getting a drug to the market and thus assuring that only the largest pharmaceutical companies could afford to develop new drugs of any significance.

Most of us realize that some regulation of drugs by government at some level is obviously necessary, particularly as to safety. But the current level of red tape, along with the requirement to prove effectiveness prior to marketing, by raising costs to astronomical levels -- now variously estimated between $250 and $500 million per new drug -- has effectively eliminated competition and established a virtual monopoly for the large "legitimate" drug cartel. Add to this the oppressive nature of the present-day regulatory apparatus of the FDA and its attempted elimination of all competitive and/or alternative methodologies and an imperious corporate state can be seen to be emerging.

THE ROCKEFELLER-I.G. FARBEN ALLIANCE

Beginning early in this century, if not even before, secret alliances were made between the chemical giants of Europe, especially I.G. Farben in Germany, and oil magnates of the US such as the enormously wealthy and unscrupulous John D. Rockefeller and his heirs. The basic element of the chemical monopoly in Europe was the same as that of the oil monopoly in the West -- *crude oil*. Nearly all synthetic drugs and most chemicals are developed from some type of petroleum base or "petrochemicals." Hence the interdependence between the oil and drug industries and the international nature of these alliances.

Quoting from Culbert's *Medical Armageddon*:

> *The discovery of oil, followed by the development of the internal combustion engine, represented steps 1 and 2 in the creation of a vast global enterprise, which, by the early 1940's, was both the largest industrial corporation in Europe and the largest chemical company in the world, with tentacles extending throughout the globe.*
>
> *In the USA, the Farben combine came to own outright or have a substantial interest in some of the best-known names in the American pharmaceutical industry, some of which were already international in scope (American I. G. Chemical, Lederle Laboratories, Sterling Drug, Winthrop Chemical, Hoffman LaRoche, Bristol Myers, Squibb and Sons Pharmaceutical, for example).* **(1)**

The author goes on to point out that the I.G. Farben tentacles extended to covert alliances with many of the well-known names in American chemical, pharmaceutical and other industries, such as Abbott Laboratories, Alcoa, Borden, Carnation, Ciba-Geigy, Dow Chemicals, DuPont, Eastman, Kodak, Monsanto Chemical and Proctor and Gamble, to name a few. There are also ties to automotive, rubber and major oil companies, such as Ford, General Motors, Firestone, General Tire, Goodyear, U.S. Rubber, Standard Oil, Shell, Taxaco, Union Oil, Richfiield, Sinclair Oil and Gulf Oil, plus hundreds of others.

None of the foregoing is intended to slander or disparage any of the fine products produced by these companies, many of which have enhanced greatly the quality of life for all of us in this country and others throughout the world. These associations are brought out here to point out the tremendous international scope and power of the top figures in these large corporate aggregations, but this is not meant to cast any reflection on the thousands of good people who produce their products.

A more detailed analysis of this enormous concentration of economic power can be found in *World Without Cancer* by G. Edward Griffin. In this monumental work, Griffin brings out the fact that it was I.G. Farben that provided the main financial backing for Adolf Hitler and his rise to power in Germany, showing the political clout of this conglomerate in the 1930s and the unsavory nature of that clout. But the interests of this huge consortium were not limited to Nazi Germany, since, through their ties to international banking, they supported Stalinist Russia as well.

In the 1920s, I.G. Farben secured agreement with the Rockefeller oil monopoly, establishing, among other things, a joint effort to develop synthetic rubber from petroleum products. When Farben carried out an apparent surrender of its holdings in 1962, Rockefeller interests then inherited an enormous amount of the world's pharmaceutical and other business. **(1)**

In *World Without Cancer*, Griffin notes:

*The Rockefeller entry into the pharmaceutical field is more concealed, however, than in most other categories of industry . . . One [reason] is the fact that, for many years before World War II, Standard Oil had a continuing cartel agreement not to enter into the broad field of chemicals except as a partner with I.G. Farben which, in turn, agreed not to compete in oil . . . Because of the unpopularity of Farben in this country and the need to camouflage its American holdings, Standard had concealed even its partnership interests in chemical firms behind a maze of false and dummy accounts. The Rockefellers' Chase Manhattan Bank, however, has always been the principal stock registrar for Farben-Rockefeller enterprises such as Sterling Drug, Olin Corporation, American Home products, and General Analine and Film. When Farben's vast holdings in the USA were finally sold in 1962, the Rockefeller group was the dominant force in carrying out the transaction. **(2)***

Various attempts at "trust-busting" have been made by the US government, including the apparent breaking up of Standard Oil in 1911, supposedly ending its monopoly. But the actual result was that the Rockefellers, through myriads of dummy trusts and hidden ownerships, by 1971 had outright control of 322 companies, including many foreign oil investments. **(3)**

The Rockefeller/Farben influence, of course, has not been limited to petro-chemicals and pharmaceuticals, but has extended into banking and financial institutions, as noted by Griffin and others. In 1933, legislation was attempted, because of growing public concern, to curb the growth of this huge concentration of economic power. Again the result was more window dressing than meaningful change. All that really happened was that the banking monopoly was reorganized and actually expanded through powerful forces directing and manipulating the very legislation which was supposed to correct the problem.

It is not the purpose or the scope of this book to delve deeply into the machinations of the international banking cartel or its many ramifications and influences on all of our lives. To go into detail on this subject would require several volumes of equal or greater size, and this has been covered extensively in other books. **(4,5,6)**

To me, the salient point in all of this is that the growth of greater and greater monopolies has not only been allowed by government to continue, but has been actually fostered by that same government. It must be remembered that without government protection, monopolies could not exist. The interests of the Rockefellers and others of the super-rich have not been confined to the various industries briefly listed in this book, but extends to government as well. The influence exerted by these "aristocrats" on our government has been enormous, through the placement of individuals beholden to Rockefeller interests into important positions, including, but certainly not limited to, top positions in the FDA.

The Rockefeller-dominated Council on Foreign Relations (CFR) has had, over most of this century, an inordinate influence on the foreign and domestic policies of the United States. While the CFR is not officially an agency of the US government, this "fraternity" includes many if not most of the influential members of the *elite* of American society, both in and out of government, including the titans of the electronic and print media.

It has been stated that no American president from either major political party over the past 80 or more years could have been elected without the approval and sanction of the CFR. Many well-documented books have made a convincing case for this seemingly unbelievable contention. **(4,7)**

Industrial monopolies or cartels cannot flourish in a truly free marketplace or in the political climate of limited government. They must make certain that laws are passed which secure their position against all competition. Evidence of this has been presented throughout this book, at least as related to the pharmaceutical division of this consortium. Many of our citizens have been led to believe by the mass media that our government has been *protecting* us from giant cartels, and in a truly limited and representative government this would be the case. However, as we have observed government expand its power and influence, we see that the opposite is true, and that bigger government begets bigger monopolies.

Throughout the history of the cartels, these monstrosities have been found to be the secret promoters of more and more power in government, whether in this country or abroad.

They were the hidden backers of Hitler's Nazi Germany, of Mussolini's Fascist Italy, and of the Bolsheviks' Communist Russia. Wherever totalitarian power arises, the super-rich and their gigantic cartels can be found operating behind the scenes. Unfortunately, this is no less so in the United States as we see the CFR and its allies exerting more and more influence on our political institutions.

Our "experts" in the media have been extoling the virtues of socialism over the years, while (rightly) telling us about the horrors of Nazism and Fascism. The real truth of the matter is that socialism, by whatever name, and however lofty its stated goals, has the same end result -- namely, more power at the top -- which inevitably grows into total power, or totalitarianism. Those we regard as authorities on the subject seem conveniently to forget or neglect to mention that the coined word "Nazi" actually stood for the National *Socialist* German Workers party.

Again, quoting G.E. Edward Griffin in *World Without Cancer:*

> *At first glance, many persons cannot understand why the "super rich" so often are found in support of socialism or socialist measures. To the uninitiated, it would appear that these would be the people with the most to lose. But under socialism -- or any other form of big government -- there is no competition and there is no free enterprise, a goal much to be desired if one not only is operating a cartelized industry but also happens to have powerful political influence "at the top." This way, one can make larger profits and be part of the ruling class as well. These people do not fear the progressive taxation scheme that oppresses the middle class, for their political influence enables them to set up elaborate tax-exempt foundations to preserve and multiply their*

great wealth with virtually no tax at all.   Which is why monopolists can never be true capitalists. **(2)**

The motivation of the monopolists we have been discussing throughout this book is therefore not limited to money and greed alone, but includes another important driving force -- power.   One of the Rockefellers made the admission, during a political campaign, that with all the great wealth he and his brother had, the only thing they had left to aspire to was political power.

Throughout all recorded history, there have always been certain men who have had an insatiable appetite for power over other men, and this aspect of human nature (in certain individuals) has not really changed over the centuries.   What has changed is the methodology used to attain that power, which has become more subtle, more devious, and more sophisticated.   Modern would-be masters stay behind the scenes, having benefited from the mistakes of the tyrants of old such as Genghis Khan, who failed using the direct approach to world conquest.

The ultimate goal of all totalitarians, by definition of course, is total control.   Not too long ago we heard former President Bush boasting about being a part of what he openly referred to as "The New World Order."   Since Bush's public pronouncement, our politicians have been more careful not to be too candid about showing their support for world government, which, of course, by its very nature must be total or totalitarian.

Much criticism has been leveled recently at those few authors who have dared to bring forth this information about what have been labeled "conspiracy theories of history" by the mass media.   But it must be remembered that the ownership and control of the major TV networks, along with those of the most prestigious news magazines and newspaper chains in this country, come under the pervasive influence of the CFR and the cartels we have been discussing.

It must also be remembered that the number-one job of all conspirators is to convince their victims that no conspiracy exists.   If these activities, carried out to the detriment of the ordinary citizen and deliberately concealed from his knowledge, do not come under the definition of conspiracy, then I have been using the wrong dictionaries (Webster's, American Heritage, Random House Thesaurus, etc.)

Authors and opinion-molders throughout the full range of the political spectrum have voiced concern about this concentration of power, both economic and political, in the hands of a few.   The reader is encouraged to explore as many as possible of the references given here, as well as others on the subject -- not just to take my word for it or that of co-author Culbert -- as to the truth of every statement made on this subject, as well as all other subjects included in this book.

It is the opinion of these authors that our efforts in exposing this threat to our liberties -- health-related and otherwise -- should be aimed at the US Congress, particularly the House of Representatives, directing our representatives to reduce the power and reach of government, particularly its constitutionally questionable agencies such as the FDA, as well as the influence of the cartels.

This will be an enormous task because these syndicates have become deeply entrenched over many years, and have developed an inordinate influence and control over both of our major political parties and our sources of information, medical and otherwise. The FDA must be taken to task and made accountable, and much of its arbitrary and unconstitutional power removed, especially with regard to its protectionism and unjustified attacks on medical alternatives.

REFERENCES

1.   Culbert, M., *Medical Armageddon*. San Diego, CA: C and C Communications, 1995.

2.   Griffin, G.E., World Without Cancer. Westlake Village, CA: American Media, 1974.

3.   Hoffman, W. David, Report on a Rockefeller. New York: Lyle Stuart, 1971.

4.   Allen, G., *The Rockefeller File*. Seal Beach, CA: '76 Press, 1976.

5.   Josephson, M., *The Robber Barons*, New York: Harcourt Brace, 1934.

6.   Flynn, J.T., *God's Gold: The Story of Rockefeller and His Times*, New York: Harcourt Brace, 1932.

7.   Perloff, J., *The Shadows of Power: The Council on Foreign Relations and The American Decline.* Appleton, WI: Western Islands, 1988.

APPENDIX

LABORATORY TESTING

Live Blood Analysis or Darkfield Microscopy

Many "alternative" practitioners now utilize the darkfield microscope in evaluating the nutritional and immune status of their patients.

Developed in Germany, this uniquely designed microscope was originally used to detect spirochetes, the causative organisms of syphilis, in the blood. This instrument was used extensively in this country and throughout the world in the 1930s and 1940s in establishing the diagnosis of syphilis, at the time the most devastating of the sexually transmitted diseases.

Less well-known is the much wider application of the darkfield microscope which allows us to evaluate disease tendencies, multiple vitamin and mineral deficiencies as well as the status of the immune system.

Meticulous study and a lifetime of research by professor Gunther Enderlein of Germany laid the groundwork for our present knowledge of this fascinating field. Enderlein found microscopic organisms which were inherent in the human which, he theorized, were capable of undergoing "pleomorphism" or changes in shape, size and other characteristics. These were not organisms which came from outside the body, but were present at birth and throughout life. Depending upon the "terrain" or the condition of the body -- acidity, alkalinity, state of nutrition and other factors -- these organisms could profoundly affect one's health, being able to become friend or foe depending upon the nutritional status of the host. The controversial work of Enderlein has been confirmed by others, including the Canadian scientist Gaston Naessans.

From the practical standpoint, the darkfield microscope enables us to determine the immune status of our patients as well as establishing to some degree the nature and extent of their disease.

Among other things, by being able to look at live blood, we are able to observe the level of activity of white blood cells.

As we have seen (Chapter VI) the white blood cells are our first line of defense against cancer and many other diseases. The activity of these blood cells can be observed only in their live state and this can be done only with the darkfield microscope.

A standard blood count, as done routinely in the conventional laboratory, is carried out on a dried blood smear which has been treated with a chemical laboratory, is carried out on a dried blood smear which has been treated with a chemical fixative and then stained, enhancing the appearance of the blood cells but rendering them lifeless. Thus no observation can be made as to the *viability* of these cells, or their activity and effectiveness as defenders, by looking at a stained blood smear.

This is not to say that the standard blood count as done in most laboratories is not useful in evaluating patients. My office uses these blood counts routinely.

But for our purposes the darkfield or live blood examination provides us with a great deal more useful information. This includes not only the level of activity of the white blood cells but other indicators of the status of the immune system as well.

By means of new and improved technology, including a TV monitor, patients are able to visualize their own blood as the technician is explaining the details of the analysis. With subsequent live blood analysis, we are able to follow the patient's progress, and the patient is also able to observe this progress on the monitor, thus providing encouragement and re-enforcement of the patient's positive attitude toward his or her program.

It has been my observation that when patients are active and informed participants in their health care, the chances of positive results are greatly improved.

As noted in some of the case histories at the beginning of this book, it is often possible to detect subtle changes in the patient's immune system early enough to make the necessary corrections before clinical symptoms or manifestations of cancer or other diseases appear.

Thus the darkfield microscope is a useful tool for prevention as well as for following the progress of treatment. having used the live blood examinations for about 15 years, I have found darkfield microscopy to be most helpful in caring for my patients. Of course this is still just one test and should be used along with other testing, including conventional laboratory studies.

Anti-Malignin Antibody Test

A test for cancer antibodies has been developed in recent years called the Anti-Malignin Antibody in Serum or AMAS test, developed by a private laboratory in Boston called ONCOLAB, under the direction of Dr. Samuel Bogoch. This blood test determines the presence of antibodies to malignin, a substance present in patients with cancer. Its accuracy has been established to be 95% on first determination and over 99% on repeat testing. **(1)**

For many years there has been a crying need for a sensitive and accurate test for cancer -- especially the early or hidden cases. We hear and read much about the importance of *early detection* of cancer. Now we have at our disposal a simple, non-invasive and relatively inexpensive test for such detection early on, or possibly even before clinical manifestations appear. There is substantial evidence of a high frequency of undetected cancer, illustrated, for example, by the common finding of previously unsuspected cancer of the prostate at autopsy. **(2)**

Unfortunately, at this point the AMAS test is not able to determine the location or area of involvement with the cancer. However, possibly in the future, radioactive labelling of the anti-malignin antibody may provide such localization of early malignant changes. **(3)** On the other hand, if one accepts the premises and postulations presented in this book -- namely, that, given the proper raw materials and providing a favorable terrain, the body has the ability to eliminate cancer -- the localization of tumors at a very early stage becomes less important.

In England, the AMAS test is being used more and more extensively for early detection of breast cancers, replacing the less reliable mammogram.

Another test for cancer is the CEA (Cancer Embryonic Antigen), which is another method of measuring cancer antigens, but which is less specific, much less consistent, and which becomes elevated late in the disease. The AMAS test, on the other hand, is much more accurate by measuring a more well-defined antibody which rises early in the disease. In some cases, the AMAS has been found to be elevated as long as two years before the clinical development or detection of cancer.

Anti-malignin antibody is the first reliable general cancer antibody to be found to indicate extent of disease and patient prognosis. This test is also useful in situations where signs and symptoms possibly point to cancer but a confirmation test is needed. Of course the AMAS or any other test alone cannot be considered as absolute confirmation of the diagnosis, but I have found this method of testing to be very useful in diagnosis as well as in following the progress of cancer patients.

An interesting, if not frustrating, aspect of this test is the reluctance of the establishment to accept it and to utilize it for cancer screening or detection, in spite of the fact that thousands of tests have been done, including a study by the prestigious Smith Kline Laboratories, confirming its accuracy. **(4)** One can only speculate as to the possibility of a more universal acceptance of the AMAS test had it been developed, say, by NIH (National Institutes of Health -- or maybe in this case, Not Invented Here.)

The use of the foregoing alternative methods of testing, of course, is not intended to exclude the use of standard laboratory tests, such as chemistry panels, blood counts, and various conventional methods of evaluating the immune system, such as T-cell quantification. These continue to have their place and are used regularly in my facility.

More information on the AMAS test can be obtained by calling 1-800-9CA-TEST.

REFERENCES

1.   Bogoch, S., *et al.*, "Early detection and monitoring of cancer with the Anti-Malignin Antibody Test." *Cancer Detect. Prev.* 18(1): 65-78, 1994.

2.   Cohen, P., *et al.*, "On the role of aging in cancer incidence: An interpretaion of the prostate cancer anomaly with implications for routine screeing." *Prostate* 6: 437-443, 1985.

3.   Bogoch, S., et al., "In vitro production of the general transformation antibody related to survival in human cancer patients: Anti-malignin antibody." *Cancer Detect. Prev.* 12: 313-320, 1988.

4.   *Protides Bio. Fluids* 31: 739-747, 1984.

PARTIAL LIST OF ALTERNATIVE PUBLICATIONS

Alternative Medicine Digest.
Future Medicine Publishing, Inc.
1640 Tiburon Blvd., Suite 2
Tiburon, CA 94920

Alternative Therapies in Health and Medicine
InnoVision Communications
101 Columbia, Aliso Viejo, CA 92656

Townsend Letter for Doctors and Patients
911 Tyler St. Port Townsend, WA 98368

The Journal of Alternative and Complementary Therapies
Mary Ann Liebert, Inc.
2 Madison Ave. Larchmont, NY 10538

Health and Healing
Julian Whitaker, MD
Phillips Publishing
7811 Montrose Rd., Potomac, MD 20854

Journal of Advancement in Medicine
ACAM, American College of Advancement in Medicine
Human Sciences Press, Inc.
233 Spring St., NY, NY 10013

Alternatives -- For the Health Conscious Individual
Dr. David Williams
Mountain Home Publishing
2700 Cummings Lane, Kerrville, TX 78028

Journal of Longevity Research
Health Quest Publications
316 California Avenue
Reno, NV 89509

The Choice
Committee for Freedom of Choice in Medicine, Inc.
1180 Walnut Avenue
Chula Vista, CA 91911

Naturally Well. Healing with the Power of Nature
Dr. Marcus Laux
Phillips Publishing Inc.
7811 Montrose Rd., Potomac, MD 20854

The Mindell Letter
Dr. Earl Mindell
Phillips Publishing Inc.
7811 Montrose Rd., Potomac, MD 20854

Health and Longevity
Robert D. Willix Jr., MD
105 West Monument St.
P.O. Box 17477
Baltimore, MD 21298

Health Revelations
Dr. Robert Atkins
P.O. Box 17097
Baltimore, MD 21298

Health Freedom News
National Health Federation
P.O. Box 688
Monrovia, CA 91016

Second Opinion
William Campbell Douglass, MD
Suite 100, 7100 Peachtree--Dunwoody Rd.
Atlanta, GA 30328

GLOSSARY

AMINO ACID: A component or "building block" required for the construction of all protein compounds. There are some 40 amino acids utilized by the body to construct its huge variety of proteins, only some 10 or 11 of these amino acids being "essential", i.e. those that the body cannot synsthesize and must obtain from food.

ANTIBODY: A protein body chemical made by B lymphocytes as part of the immune response to allergens, infectious agents, foreign chemicals and diseases such as cancer.

ANTIGENS: A foreign or disease-producing substance, which brings about a reaction by the body's immune system, consisting of the production of antibodies.

B-LYMPHOCYTES: Specialized white blood cells produced by the bone marrow, able to produce many thousands of highly specialized antibodies which counteract specific antigens or disease producing substances.

CACHEXIA: A condition of wasting of the body, consisting of loss of appetite, profound weight loss, severe weakness, and usually a breakdown of many body systems, common in terminal stages of cancer and AIDS.

CANCER: A group or cluster of body cells which have undergone degeneration and transformation to a state of uncontrolled multiplication and abnormal cell division, thought by many to have been initiated by free radical damage to the DNA of the cell.

CARCINOGEN: A substance, most often a toxic chemical, which is capable of changing a normal cell into a cancer cell.

CAROTENOIDS: A large number of vitamin and vitamin-like substances, derived from plants, including vitamin A and its precursors, most of which are colored orange, yellow or red.

CHEMOTHERAPY: Synthetic cytotoxic drugs, or combinations of drugs used in the treatment of cancer. These drugs and combinations have the capability of killing rapidly-dividing cells, such as cancer cells, but are not highly selective and thus are toxic to normal cells as well.

COENZYME: A natural substance which acts as a co-factor in a specific enzyme reaction by combining temporarily with that enzyme.

CYTOTOXIC: Any substance or combination of substances able to poison or kill cells, including both normal and abnormal cells, such as cancer cells.

CYTOKINES: Protein substances or peptides which facilitate communication between cells, usually between various types of white blood cells involved in the immune system.

DNA: Desoxyribonucleic acid. The helical, double-stranded molecule in the nucleus of the cell making up the genetic material and establishing the nature of all offspring of that cell.

EFFUSION: An excessive amount of fluid in a body cavity, such as the abdominal cavity or chest cavity, outside the lung.

FREE RADICAL: A free floating particle of an atom which contains an unpaired electron, and which is extremely unstable and capable of causing cell damage, including DNA damage and cell degeneration.

HOMEOPATHY: A discipline of medical practice in which symptoms of disease and combinations of symptoms are treated with tiny doses of substances and drugs which in larger or normal doses would produce the same symptoms in a healthy individual. Modern allergy treatment is based upon the principles of homeopathy.

IMMUNE SYSTEM: The complex organization of organs and functions in the body designed to defend against disease-causing substances or organisms. This includes both cellular and humoral or antibody elements of the immune system.

INTERFERON: One of a group of peptides which act as chemical messengers between different types of lymphocytes, and serve to activate specialized T-cells in fighting viral infections and cancer. Used in the conventional treatment of cancer by activating certain aspects of the immune system. Occasionally used in alternative protocols as well.

INTERLEUKINS: Another group of cell communicating peptides involved in activating macrophages as well as T-cells. Used conventionally in treating cancer.

LEUKEMIA: A malignant condition of the blood and blood-producing organs, consisting of an excessive production of white blood cells, usually accompanied by a reduction of red blood cells and platelets.

LEUKOCYTE: A white blood cell which contains a nucleus. Types of leukocytes include polymorphonuclear leukocytes or granulocytes which are mostly infection-fighters. Monocytes, eosinophiles and lymphocytes are also included among the leukocytes.

LYMPHOCYTE: A type of white blood cell or leukocyte which is involved in the defense against many diseases, including cancer. T-cells and B-cells are two types of lymphocytes.

LYMPHOKINE: A peptide or protein produced in the lymphocyte which acts as a chemical messenger allowing one lymphocyte to communicate with another. The interleukins are lymphokines.

MACROPHAGE: Literally "big eater" cells of the immune-system, found mostly in the tissues, which act as first line of defense against disease, including cancer. These cells have the ability to recognize, envelope and devour foreign substances, bacteria, viruses and cancer cells, acting as phagocytes or "eaters."

METASTASIS: The process by which cancer cells spread and/or migrate from one area of the body to another, either through the lymphatic system or the blood stream: from primary to distant sites.

MITOCHONDRIA: One or more microscopic compartments of each cell supplying all of energy for that cell. The "battery" or "batteries" of the cell.

NECROSIS: Death of cells and/or tissues, usually as a result of disease.

ONCOLOGIST: A physician with an MD degree who has specialized training in the orthodox methods of treating cancer, primarily with the use of chemotherapeutic drugs.

ONCOLOGY: The study of tumors. The science of the treatment of cancer, especially with drugs.

PEPTIDES: Two or more amino acids linked together in chains or various combination to form specialized protein substances. Longer chains of amino acids are usually referred to as polypeptides.

PERITONEUM: Abdominal cavity normally containing fluid in which intestinal tract is bathed or "floating."

PLEURAL: Referring to the normally thin space outside the lungs and within the chest cavity.

PROSTAGLANDINS: A variety of fatty acid substances produced by the body and involved in various chemical aspects of the immune response.

SARCOMA: A type of cancer arising in connective tissue, bone, cartilage or muscle, as opposed to carcinomas which arise in glandular or epithelial tissues.

T-LYMPHOCYTES: Specialized lymphocytes which are under the influence and direction of the thymus. T-cells are sub-divided into "helper" T-cells, "suppressor" T-cells, and NK or natural killer cells, each carrying out its specialized function.

TERMINAL: Referring to the irreversible or end stage of a fatal disease such as cancer.

THYMUS GLAND: The small gland beneath the breast bone which is considered an important controlling factor of immune function, responsible for the maturation and the behavior of all T-cells.

VITAMIN: A naturally occurring food substance, required by the body for a number of functions, water- or fat-soluble, not synthesized by the body but required from outside food sources, a lack of which will result in a specific deficiency disease. Many vitamins now are recognized as being inter-dependent and capable of preventing a wide variety of diseases.